gluten-free girl

gluten-free girl

HOW I FOUND

THE FOOD THAT

LOVES ME BACK...

& HOW YOU CAN, TOO

shauna james ahern

BICENTENNIAL
1807
WILEY
2007
BICENTENNIAL

John Wiley & Sons, Inc.

Published by John Wiley & Sons, Inc., Hoboken, New Jersey
Published simultaneously in Canada

Design and composition by Navta Associates, Inc.

The information contained in this book is not intended to serve as a replacement for professional medical advice. Any use of the information in this book is at the reader's discretion. The author and the publisher specifically disclaim any and all liability arising directly or indirectly from the use or application of any information contained in this book. A health care professional should be consulted regarding your specific situation.

For general information about our other products and services, please contact our Customer Care Department within the United States at (800) 762-2974, outside the United States at (317) 572-3993 or fax (317) 572-4002.

Wiley also publishes its books in a variety of electronic formats. Some content that appears in print may not be available in electronic books. For more information about Wiley products, visit our web site at www.wiley.com.

ISBN: 978-0470-13730-7

Printed in the United States of America

10   9   8   7   6   5   4   3   2   1

For Danny, whose love feeds me.

contents

acknowledgments

You know it's a good party when everyone is in the kitchen, leaning against the countertops with wineglasses dangling from fingertips, talking and laughing, hands reaching for another bite of food. There is nothing I like more than making food for hours, then watching everyone sigh with pleasure at the first bite.

This party is a particular celebration.

Dear Merida comes up the steps bearing a spiced lentil salad, ringed with slices of lemon. Sharon—up from Los Angeles for the weekend—is laughing as she reaches for another homemade potato chip. Cindy and Gabe, in from New York, talk animatedly in the corner, their eyes wide. Tita unwraps the casserole she has brought from Vashon Island, as John stands by her, a little shy with all these people. Daniel arrives bearing dahlias from his garden, and Jeff holds two bottles of Washington State wine. Amal is eyeing the lemon sorbet. Seis and Pia are standing in the living room, talking with Lisa and Mane, while Reina and King play with my blue exercise ball. Bill and Carol are beaming at their daughter's photographs on my wall, while Monica meanders over for more coffee. Molly brandishes her homemade applesauce with a meringue topping, and Brandon has brought another skillet he found at Goodwill. Dorothy made roasted red pepper soup. Paul and Amy brought a platter of caprese salad: slices of fresh mozzarella, rounds of beefsteak tomatoes, and basil from the garden. Françoise arrives, and the entire room lightens with the energy she shepherds in behind her, along with Adriaan, Camille, and Selene. Stephanie, Deb, and Hortensia arrive from the restaurant, at the end of their shift. Quinn and Pete talk about fishing, while they portion out the gravalax with dill. Mary McKillop brings potato salad and bad news of the Mariners' latest loss. Tara grins and dives into the mixed green salad with goat cheese. Julie—eager for another conversation about food—asks each person about his or her favorite meal.

No one ever writes a book alone, even though the act of writing is solitary. All these people, gathered in my home, have helped me produce the words you hold in your hands.

And they are there, that Sunday, the day of my "Hey, the book is finally done. Let's celebrate!" party, because they are my friends. But also because each one has added some essential taste to my life, and a particular sustenance to my existence, during those long months of writing.

After a couple hours of eating, drinking, and telling stories, we gather in the kitchen together. I pour each person a tall glass of sparkling wine—dry, with a touch of sweetness—and we raise our glasses to toast all those who could not be in the kitchen that day.

To Marguerite, who mentioned a gluten-free friend of hers while we bobbed in the pool.

To Anne and Rick, who were excellent first readers and a vital connection.

To Rachael, my fairy god–blogger, who arranged for Le Creuset to send me an entire set of cookware.

To all the friends and faculty members at the Sitka Fine Arts Camp, who made me feel supported as a writer, and helped me to see I that should pursue this love.

To all my former students, who allowed me to be part of their lives. By teaching them how to write, I taught myself what I wanted to say.

To Gwen, at *Allergic Living*, who gave me my first magazine column.

To every gluten-free food producer, cooking his or her heart out to make food safe and accessible for all of us. (Another toast to those who sent me food for free.)

To Bette Hagman, for paving the way, and to Dr. Peter Green at Columbia for educating us.

To the farmers, who have grown the food we are eating.

To the restaurateurs in Seattle, who go to great lengths to feed me, safely.

To Jamie Oliver, Julia Child, Alice Waters, and Judy Rodgers.

To Kate at Accidental Hedonist for establishing the Food Blog Awards.

To all my fellow food bloggers, who make me feel part of a community when I take photographs of my food.

To a few bloggers in particular: David Lebovitz, Heidi Swanson, and Clotilde Dusoulier, who believed in my blog early on and wrote the quotes for my book proposal. And to Luisa, for her tart take on all those recipes.

To Nicole Champagne, Sarah Porter, Becky Selengut, Kristin Shamordola, and Cari Trousdale, for testing recipes and offering suggestions.

To Judy, Eric, and Ingrid at SeeSaw Productions, who believed I was worth following around with a camera.

To Stacey Glick, at Dystel and Goderich, the best literary agent in the world, a dream come true.

To Christel Winkler, the most incredible editor I could imagine, who supported my words through deep cuts and impossible deadlines and more cuts.

To everyone at Wiley, who took a chance on this first-time author.

To all my readers, for leaving comments and suggestions, feedback and questions, and who have made me feel that my words were worthwhile.

To Dana and Elliott, for bringing such joy and laughter into my life.

To Andy, my brother and best friend all my life.

To Mom and Dad, who made me, and continue to make me happy that I'm alive.

After all these toasts, we are almost out of wine. The light is fading in the sky outside. But we have one more toast to make, perhaps the most important one. With the last drops left, we raise our glasses high. To the Chef, who is standing by the stove, misty eyed and proud. My love, my love, I could not have done this without you.

1

a brand-name childhood

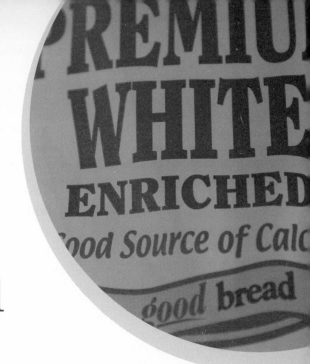

I grew up in a processed-foods generation, raised on white flour and white sugar. When my friends and I talk about the food we ate growing up, we only talk about brand names. Cap'n Crunch. Diet Coke. Cheetos. We were brand loyal almost before we were born. I don't remember fresh ingredients or creative meals. I remember jingles.

When I walk into the kitchen after school, I find a plethora of choices waiting for me. On the orange countertops, a loaf of Wonder Bread, soft slices spilling out from the plastic wrapper. Should I make a grilled cheese sandwich with American cheese, cloaked in more plastic? Or a fried bologna sandwich slathered with margarine?

When I open the avocado green drawers, I find boxes of Cracker Jack, piles of Astro Pops, cans of Pringles, and enough Abba-Zaba bars to keep my teeth busy for days.

In the wood-paneled cupboards, lined up in neat rows, sit stiff cardboard boxes of Hamburger Helper, little packets of Top Ramen, and cans of Campbell's soup. Plus, there is always the cereal: boxes of Frosted Flakes, Lucky Charms, and an almost-full box of Grape-Nuts in the back. For a snack, I could just grab a pint-size cereal, the one that comes in six-packs—a kid's idea of a party—and eat it right out of the box. Naaah.

So I move to the fridge. Oscar Mayer bacon sits in the bottom drawer. Sometimes, when I'm hungry in my head, and I want to get back at my mother, I think about nibbling on strips of raw bacon. It probably has enough nitrites to protect me from salmonella. But I don't. Instead, I eye the leftover tuna-noodle casserole in a Pyrex dish. A carton of orange juice and a tub of cottage cheese. Gross—who wants those? The only fruit in the house—some mushy Red Delicious apples, months away from the tree, the too-red color bleeding into the white flesh—sits moldering in the back. And on the door, a bottle of vile-tasting worm medicine, which my mother insists I take daily since my stomach is always grumbling. She's convinced that I have a tapeworm. I close the door.

There is always something in the freezer. When I open it with a flourish, the cold steam billows outward. My mother, perpetually panicked about our safety, turns up the knob in the refrigerator to the highest setting, ensuring that nothing spoils. Some mornings, I have to break a thin layer of ice on the milk before I pour it in my bowl. Sometimes, I put my head in the freezer, just to escape the heat. This is Los Angeles, land of constant sunshine. Whenever I open the freezer door, I find packaged food: cartons of frozen pizza, tubs of Rocky Road ice cream, and a few stray boxes of frozen spinach.

But the summer I turned ten, I knew what I would find in the freezer, and I always went straight for it. Stuffed in among the other foods, in piles of crinkly packets, was my fix: Clark bars. We had hundreds of Clark bars slotted into the spaces of our freezer that year.

My parents had been on a game show called *Let's Make a Deal*, where people dressed in outlandish costumes and thronged the auditorium, stretching out their hands to be noticed by the host, in the desperate hope of being on television. My parents—so I am told—dressed up in the following attire. My mother wore a pink hat, to which she had somehow attached a head full of pickles. She held up a sign made with magic markers: I'D BE PICKLED PINK TO BE ON THIS SHOW. My father, a college writing instructor, wore his favorite golf hat, to which he had stapled half a head of iceberg lettuce. His sign? LETTUCE MAKE A DEAL.

They were chosen. However, they faltered on the first assignment, a bidding war with other contestants. If they had won, they could have gone on to the individual competition, where they might have won a Pontiac car or a new Maytag washer. But they lost on the first question, in which they had to guess the price of a bottle of high-quality champagne. Never having drunk any in their lives, they guessed ten dollars.

That's why we had a freezer full of Clark bars. It was their consolation prize. Every day, I ate the cloyingly sweet, chocolate-flavored concoction, with the crumbles of peanut butter dulled inside, the crumbs tumbling onto my lap as I sat in front of the television. I ate one, not feeling well, but never knowing anything different. Life might have been confusing, but I had junk food to tide me over.

This was the food of my childhood.

I was not the only one eating this way. If you want to set a room full of *Brady Bunch*–generation adults talking, ask them about the cereals they ate as kids. "Count Chocula!" someone shouted once, after a twenty-minute heated discussion of Honeycomb, Chex, and Cocoa Pebbles. At the sound of the name, this group of lawyers, engineers, and teachers turned ten years old again. "Oh, my God, Count Chocula!" We each had our favorite brands, and the daring among us would mix them: a bit of Trix, some Life Cereal, and more Alpha-Bits. Sugar and more sugar—we just craved that sweetened milk and enriched white flour. My friend Paul says that his most vivid food memory was going to a friend's house, where he discovered that they ate Raisin Bran for breakfast. Pouting, he put three spoonfuls of sugar in his bowl before he could even stomach the taste. We were raised on the sugary stuff, almost all of us.

My friends with the mothers who insisted on hot cereal and grainy flakes felt deprived because they couldn't eat what everyone else in the United States ate. No one my age remembers eating whole-grain bread as children, except for the one who was raised in Berkeley. I have a friend whose mother woke up early every morning to make three loaves of white bread from scratch, just so her seven children could eat warm, homemade goodness for lunch. But still, my friend felt ostracized at school, because she didn't have Wonder Bread in her lunch box. Being normal meant having that squishy white bread.

An entire generation was raised to believe that cooking meant opening a box, ripping off plastic wrap, or adding water. The television told us what to eat, and we paid attention. But after a lifetime of grabbing burgers from fast-food joints and eating in the backseat of our cars, we are a cooking-illiterate generation. We're fascinated by food, and we know we should be healthier, but we don't know how. We only know how to tear open a package and stick it in the microwave.

We were a typical American family: baby boomer parents with Gen X kids, living in the suburbs of Los Angeles. We lived in the land of shrink-wrapped plastic and the endless vapidity that comes from desperately wanting to look good, all the time. We were smiling children, both stars in school. Dad was the coach of the soccer team; Mom was the head of the PTA. Mom organized potlucks at school and made class cookbooks with recipes for chili casserole with crushed corn chips, mimeographed in smeary blue ink.

We were not out of the norm of American society.

We also really weren't that normal.

When I was seven, my mother plunged into agoraphobia, which kept her trapped in the house with her fears. She kept us trapped there with her. She feared anything different, an almost visceral reaction to anything too weird. Everything needed to be just like what she saw on television. Like the rest of America.

We ate what she thought the rest of the country did. No funky grains or odd vegetables. No "ethnic" foods, including that strange "Oriental" cuisine. She cooked breaded and fried food. We ate our peanut butter and jelly sandwiches on bleached white bread. Day-Glo orange macaroni and cheese out of a box. Green beans from a can, clotted with cream of mushroom soup and crusted with fried onions.

Not only did we eat TV dinners in my stuffy little house—with soggy fried chicken, mashed potatoes with a fake yellow butter substitute, and that volcanically hot cherry dessert—but we also dutifully ate them on our individual TV trays while watching *Happy Days*.

I remember feeling always vaguely unwell, slightly run-down, and easily tired, even at ten years old. Bookish by nature, I became even more so by practice, since my body always wanted to lie down. I caught every bug that went through my school. As soon as I hit puberty, I suffered from hormonal problems.

At best, I felt just okay. I never knew what it would be like to feel *good*.

Sometimes, I felt horribly unwell: wheezing chest, headaches, and fevers; desperate fatigue. I developed pneumonia six times in my life, nearly dying once. If it wasn't pneumonia, it was bronchitis, my throat constricted, my chest squeezed tight. Breathing in too deeply—more than half-hearted pants—brought prickles of pain deep in my lungs.

At the time, my parents blamed my poor health on the smog. Brown gunk lay thick over the obscured San Bernardino hills, only twenty miles from our front door. Some days, Dr. George Fishbeck, the wacky weatherman on KABC, advised us not to go outside at all, unless it was absolutely necessary. In my family, it was hardly ever necessary. We lived in our little cave, together and alone, eating junk food and staying in separate corners as long as we could.

When I was a sophomore in high school, I developed an inexplicable, fiery pain in my belly, horrible searing cramps, unbearable lassitude, and an inability to eat the prepackaged foods that lay before me. My mother, concerned as always that I was dying, took me to the family doctor, a decrepit German man, who probably graduated from medical school before the 1929 stock market crash. He pronounced me fine. My symptoms continued.

After repeated visits, he blithely suggested I might have ovarian cancer. I was fifteen. Over the next few weeks, I endured nearly every medical test known to man, including one that forced me to live on only liquids for three days of preparation (my parents gave me warm Dr. Pepper and canned chicken broth), another with iodine dye run through my kidneys, and a barium enema X-ray.

No clear answers emerged. After the last test, one doctor informed me that the X-rays showed that my lower intestines were kinked. Clearly, it had all obviously been stress. He gave me some vague breathing techniques and sent me home. After all those tests and terror, my parents let me eat whatever my body wanted to eat—nothing but spinach, boiled chicken, and navel oranges for weeks. I tried to practice my breathing. Miraculously, I started to feel better.

No one ever mentioned celiac disease to me. I didn't even know what gluten was. At that time, anyone who avoided wheat was regarded as a bit of a freak, especially by my mother. Who wouldn't want glorious all-American food? Even in my senior year of high school, when I was dissecting a cadaver in my anatomy and physiology class and studying the intestines closely, I had no idea that white bread could ever make me sick.

It took me twenty more years to find out.

There I stood on a driveway in Malibu, sixteen years old, reading a copy of *Laurel's Kitchen*. I clutched it to me and handed the owner of the garage sale fifty cents, then tucked it under my arm so my parents couldn't see what I had bought.

Laurel's Kitchen, written by Laurel Robertson, Carol Flinders, and Bronwen Godrey, was one of the first major American books on vegetarianism. It was published in Berkeley, California, in 1976. At the time, it seemed to me that only die-hard hippies talked about eating whole foods or growing their own gardens. Maybe the original owner of that copy of *Laurel's Kitchen* had gone on a health kick, bought the book, and then tossed it aside to dive into fast food again.

In the privacy of my bedroom, I read it, chapters at a time. I read not only the recipes for whole grains and exotic-sounding Indian food but also the narrative chapters on nutrition and how to balance proteins. Mostly, I devoured the introduction, which welcomed me into the kitchens of these women as the authors baked bread meditatively, talked about politics and how to raise their families, and made everything from scratch. Their world seemed much more at peace than mine, even though they were discussing the worst perturbations of society. They were doing something about it—rebelling—by making their own food. I felt it innately—someone has it right.

I wanted to be in that kitchen.

What was I doing reading a hippie book in the suburbs of Los Angeles in 1982? I was longing for a life entirely not my own. Those were the days of feathered hair, Vans shoes, John Hughes movies, Op shorts, good Michael Jackson songs, Ronald Reagan, prosperity and the trickle-down theory. Greed was good—remember? I was surrounded by mass consumption, bright-white teeth, and the birth of MTV.

How well do you think blemished organic fruit sold in my neighborhood?

"What are you doing, reading that ridiculous book?" my mother asked me. "Those women don't know how to cook."

But somehow, *Laurel's Kitchen* called to me. I read it and reread it, again and again. I decided to become a vegetarian, because Laurel, Carol, and Bronwen wrote that most of mainstream America seemed to feel vaguely unwell all the time. This sounded achingly familiar to me. Since they linked this feeling to eating meat, I stopped eating the steaks that came from the grocery store in polystyrene packages and the eight greasy pieces of meat from the Oscar Mayer meat pack. (The pimento loaf wasn't much of a loss.) My younger brother decided to join me.

Mom didn't like us disdaining her food. She told us that we had to make all our own meals if we wanted something special. She insisted that I eat cottage cheese with Lawry's Seasoned Salt at every meal to make up for my drastic lack of protein. In a futile attempt to make veggie burgers, I tried to combine raw tofu, barely cooked lentils, and cottage cheese into patties. They flopped and sagged; they mostly fell into the coals. What remained tasted like soggy grit. My brother and I spat them out, and within a few weeks we were back to gobbling up the family's overcooked meat.

I bet veggie burgers didn't taste like that in Laurel's kitchen.

But I didn't give up that easily. Despite my mother's loudly spoken wishes, somewhere inside me there lived a wild food hippie who wanted to roam free, foraging for whole grains.

I began to enjoy tastes other than the prepackaged, sugary-smack treats always laid before me. Slowly, I started to learn that there was a world wider than white bread out there. That world may not have been in my parents' kitchen or in any of the stores in my Southern California town, but I was going to find it.

2

on my own

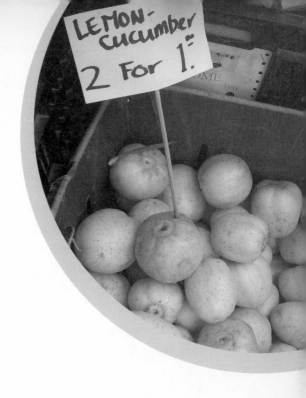

At twenty-six, I was living on a rural island off Seattle, surrounded by former hippies who had been cooking with whole foods and funky grains for decades. Finally in my own apartment, with a brand-new kitchen, I returned to my vegetarian urges of a decade previous. Since I was a high school English teacher, and living on an island bereft of single men, I had hours of time to follow my passion for food. One Saturday morning, I wandered into a small farmers' market on the island: three or four booths of people selling the zucchini they had grown in their backyards. I took the fresh vegetables home to experiment with stir-fries and salads other than iceberg with bottled blue cheese dressing. For the first time in my life, I began to truly taste what vegetables had to offer. I wanted more. One Saturday afternoon, I spent nearly an entire day making mushroom stock from scratch. The next day, I made a wild mushroom soup with sherry and cream. Hours later, I took my first sip and nearly fell on the floor. I can still taste it today, fifteen years later.

Every December, I turned out thick sugar cookies, iced in rich buttercream frosting, in quaint shapes of Christmas. Eventually, I could turn out a batch of exquisite cookies in half an hour flat. There'd be flour in my hair and bits of dough on the floor, but the plate piled high with cookies emptied quickly, leaving only green sprinkles.

Looking back on it now, I realize what I was doing those years. I was learning how to cook. With no one else to teach me, and no one else to feed, I had the time and inclination to play and taste, make mistakes, and come up with my recipes. I began eating well for the first time in my life.

After years on my little island, I moved to another island on the other side of the country.

When I moved to New York City, just after I turned thirty, I was astonished to find that I had to go out to meet friends. With every block stuffed with interesting restaurants, I never lacked for choice. But I had grown accustomed to having people over for dinner nearly every Friday night. In New York, however, not many people threw dinner parties. Why? New Yorkers don't cook. I should qualify that statement. In Queens and Brooklyn, the Bronx and Staten Island, there are Italian families still making pasta from scratch, Greek grandmothers spending all day rolling dolmas by hand, mothers from the Dominican Republic drinking *café con leches* while grating fresh tubers to make *pasteles,* and firemen making vast pots of chili for their crew. However, in Manhattan—and particularly on the Upper West Side, where I was living—people my age simply didn't cook. They ate out for every meal, even if breakfast meant an egg sandwich from the corner bodega.

This lack of home cooking was why many grocery stores were depressing places: the produce wilted and saggy ("It's like Slovenia, 1956," I always used to joke), the aisles gray from broken fluorescent lights. The independently wealthy could afford to do all their shopping at Zabar's, but most of those people still didn't cook. They nibbled and sampled, relying on prepackaged food. Knowing the right restaurant was a sign of your social standing. Cooking was for grandmothers.

However, going out to meet friends for dinner is how I first tasted authentic Indian food on 6th Street, garlicky Italian meals downtown, and crispy potato knishes from Yonah Schimmel's, all for the first time. Everything revolved around food, but someone else was always making it for me.

Eventually, my hands and mind couldn't stand it any longer. (Neither could my wallet.) I started cooking again.

My apartment in New York City was in an old building, with high ceilings and an enormous kitchen. I threw dinner parties. One Thanksgiving, I spontaneously invited over four friends who were stuck in the city. Why not host a real Thanksgiving dinner, with turkey and stuffing and pumpkin pie? When each of my friends sheepishly brought along an unexpected friend, I welcomed them all. What is better than a kitchen full of people, waiting to be fed? "But will you have enough food?" they asked. I had braved a ten-block walk from Gristedes, with six plastic bags of food on each arm, in a biting snowstorm the night before, just to ensure that I would have a homemade feast for my friends. We ate long through the evening—talking about our favorite meals and mishaps with food—and still had enough leftovers for cold turkey sandwiches at midnight.

I had to call the Butterball hotline Thanksgiving morning, just like millions of Americans, to figure out exactly how long I should cook the turkey. The stuffing made us chew a little too long to call it good. The edges of the pumpkin piecrust were slightly burnt. None of that mattered. It was my first Thanksgiving meal, and people were happy to be eating.

There was also a brief stint in London, living in a mansion off Hampstead Heath with a wealthy family. There, I ate fabulous food every night, made with the most expensive ingredients in the world, and prepared by a series of personal chefs. I discovered high-quality olive oil, mushroom risottos, and peppery arugula. I swam in a surfeit of truffles, caviar, and champagne. But I still wasn't doing the cooking myself. Believe it or not, I missed standing in front of the stove, stirring.

By the time I returned to Seattle to live, everything zinged on my tongue and woke up my senses. I still didn't feel that well, but at least everything finally had a vibrant taste: the sharp smell of ginger filling my nose, the tang of garlic attacking my tongue. The world felt wider, and mine at the same time.

On a Friday night in February, my three best girlfriends and I sat in one of our favorite restaurants in Seattle, hoisting watermelon cosmos and singing out our laughter. My job, as a writing teacher at a private arts school, fulfilled me most days. After years of wandering the world and not knowing where home was, I felt at peace with the green trees and spaciousness of Seattle. My friends were loving, funny, and growing in legion. I felt I was doing something good in the world.

But physically, life had been hard. Something felt wrong. Although I am naturally ebullient, I lagged behind everyone else in energy by the end of the day. My first winter in Seattle, I caught pneumonia. Again. My second winter in Seattle, I had abdominal surgery for a large fibroid tumor, which left me enervated. The third winter, I was nearly killed in a car accident. The experience changed me, utterly, and I felt lucky to be alive. But being alive meant being in pain. The pain from the back injuries and the repercussions from the concussion and the crunched neck never went away. I felt continuously, crushingly tired most of the time. Headaches invaded me daily, most of them pounding by the afternoon. Every time I ate, I flushed red across my nose and down my cheeks. My joints ached when it rained. I hurt, all the time.

That night, my friends and I were celebrating the fact that I had finally shaken the nasty virus that had been circulating through the city. For weeks, I had been dragging, coughing, and trying not to complain. That night, I finally felt decent. As we waited for our seared pork chops and rotisserie chicken to arrive, we dipped slice after slice of soft, crusty bread into the olive oil and balsamic vinegar before us. After nearly two weeks of my being an invalid, this felt like a decadent evening on the town.

By the time I returned home, I had developed a sudden, severe sore throat. No warning. No anticipatory shivers or gulps. Within fifteen minutes, I had to hunch on the floor of the shower under a hot spray of water just to keep warm. That night, I burned with a high fever.

Then, I descended. For the next six weeks, I was in nearly unbearable pain. Searing abdominal cramps, stabbing pains in the stomach, and a massive tenderness on my left flank—they grew worse every day. I returned to different doctors, hoping for relief, or at least some answers, but neither arrived. I slept eighteen hours a day. I missed weeks of school, the winter slipping into spring without my noticing. One day, a month into this illness, I could no longer huddle under the blanket on my couch. I had to go outside. I gingerly entered the spring air and walked to the bakery down the block, then sat on the front steps of my house, eating handfuls of the warm olive loaf I had purchased, welcoming the sun on my face. Afterward, I had to take a three-hour nap.

There was a trip to the emergency room, multiple visits to multiple doctors' offices, two ultrasounds, and two CAT scans. Then came chest X-rays, a colonoscopy and endoscopy on the same day, and more blood drawn than I could measure. Through it all loomed the possibility of kidney stones, colon cancer, stomach ulcers, endometriosis, and ovarian cancer. Every test came back negative. No one understood.

The strangest part of it—and almost the worst—was my body's sudden attitude toward food. At first, I wasn't very hungry. After having a diminished appetite, I quickly descended into no appetite. I had never been one of those women who forgets to eat or goes a week without food after a breakup with a boyfriend. However, that spring, I did not want food. In fact, after a week or so, my body simply would not accept more than half a cup of food at a time. If I ate any more, I grew violently nauseated, and my stomach started lurching with pain beneath my hands. I stopped eating much at all. I stuck to soft, easy foods—crackers, packaged puddings, Popsicles, and commercial chicken broth. An older friend of mine made me homemade bread, loaf after loaf, and I ate it in small hunks. After every ten bites, I had to take a nap.

Then, I was repulsed by food. The sight of it, the smell of it, made me physically ill. I forced myself to eat at least a jar of baby food a day, since I had lived weeks without a vegetable at this point, and I could not seem to stomach anything else. However, my body would only let me eat the pureed sweet potatoes a few spoonfuls at a time. Other than that, and the soft bread, I could not eat anything.

One afternoon in the midst of this, my friend Monica called me from the streets of New York City. I heard the sirens behind her, the rush of the crowds. I could taste it, that city. I was supposed to be there that week, which was spring break at school. At least I didn't feel guilty about missing more work. Still, it made me sad to hear the city where I was supposed to be meeting friends in favorite restaurants, instead of eating nothing but crumbs. When Monica asked how I was doing, I told her about the absence of food. "But you love food!" she shouted. "It's huge to you. That must be harder for you mentally than physically."

She was right. I felt as though I had lost some essential part of me. Shopping for food takes me hours, normally, as I touch every contour of the red peppers and sniff the spices as I walk by. Then, the cooking: the chopping, the sautéing, the smells. Oh, and the eating. I love my food. I thrive on it, write about it, talk about it, and reminisce about it. Food has always been another language for me, one I speak well. Suddenly, I felt mute.

Finally, a colleague at work and a friend from Maine called on the same day, suggesting something I had never heard of before, celiac disease. They had both heard the same report on NPR about this little-known disease that goes undiagnosed for years, with many of the same symptoms I had been suffering. Grateful for any suggestion, I looked up the condition online. After all, I had been Googling my own diagnosis for weeks, desperate for this to end.

Celiac disease is a genetic intolerance for gluten—the elastic protein in wheat, rye, barley, triticale, kamut, and spelt—and it can damage the small intestine for years, silently, or at least in a language that most of us do not know how to recognize. People suffering from headaches dismiss it as stress, those with achy joints wonder if they are experiencing early arthritis, and women with gynecological problems blame it on their hormones. Yet, each of these conditions can be a symptom of celiac disease. For various genetic reasons, the celiac's body reads gluten as a toxin and attacks it. The antibodies go after the gluten but attack the small intestine instead, leaving it incapable of absorbing proper nutrition. At best, this leaves people feeling exhausted, anxious without knowing why, and susceptible to catching colds. Later, it can lead to colon cancer and other auto-immune disorders, such as diabetes or thyroid problems.

According to the National Institutes of Health, celiac disease is the most underdiagnosed disease in the United States. For years, medical schools taught erroneously that celiac disease was a childhood disorder, as rare as 1 in 5,000 people. A prominent doctor in Seattle told me, after my diagnosis, that he spent five minutes learning about celiac disease in medical school. According to various sources, now it is understood that 1 out of 100 Americans suffer from celiac disease. That means 2 million people in the United States should be living gluten-free. Only 3 percent of us have been diagnosed—that means millions of people floundering in pain and discomfort for decades without knowing why. That number is changing, however, as awareness of the disease grows exponentially. Eighty thousand new celiac patients are being diagnosed *every month* worldwide.

When I read all this, I felt the shivers—and it wasn't the chills leading to a fever. This felt *right*.

This was my story. Every symptom of celiac disease that I read about in my research felt eerily familiar. Once before, on the advice of a nutritionist, I had cut wheat from my diet for six weeks, and I started to feel fantastic. However, wheat being so ubiquitous in our starchy, prepackaged society, I had slipped back into consuming it again. Immediately after reading about celiac disease online, I called the office of my gastroenterologist and requested a blood test for celiac disease. The answer came back in a phone message: "Ah, that's really a long shot. It's such a rare disease. We'll talk about it in your follow-up two weeks from now." Infuriated, I made an appointment with another doctor, who drew the blood for me the next day. After having my blood drawn, I cut gluten out of my diet entirely.

By the end of the first day, I started feeling better. My stomach did not throb with pain when I ate a jar of baby food. On day two, I was able to stay awake all afternoon and eat a saucer of sautéed spinach. On the third day without gluten, I looked up and realized that my brain fog had lifted. I felt as though I had been wearing smudgy contacts and someone had just cleaned them for me. I was filled with an energy I had not experienced in years.

On day five, the physical feeling of hunger came roaring back. My body wanted food again. I was profoundly aware of the beautiful sensation of hot food sliding down my throat.

It is amazing what we take for granted.

Before the blood tests came back, I knew the answer. The science confirmed what my body told me. I had celiac disease. Finally, I understood what had been going wrong in my body—not only for those past six weeks, or the past three years, but my entire life. This diagnosis explained the mystery ailment of my adolescence. It explained all the bouts of pneumonia. It explained why, as a kid, I always felt flattened with exhaustion and unable to move. My mother had given me medicine to prevent tapeworm, but it was the gluten that had made me sick.

Celiac disease is still a bit of a mystery. Why do some people develop it as infants, upon their first feeding of wheat, and others have a sudden, acute onset as adults? Scientists are not entirely sure. Those of us who have celiac disease are genetically disposed to it, but we are not born with active celiac disease. Some scientists are now theorizing that it may be a viral infection of the gastrointestinal system that causes celiac disease to awaken in the body. I believe that is what happened to me when I was fifteen. It is clear that a trauma to the body of some sort—injury, miscarriage, or even stress—can trigger the body into full-blown celiac disease. In my case, with abdominal surgery one winter, a car accident the next, and a terrible virus in the third winter, the disease developed fully in my body, until I could no longer ignore it.

After cutting out gluten, I felt clear and energized. I realized that I had lived my entire life without ever meeting my real self. Now, I was finally well. I was free—finally, wonderfully free.

All I had to do to heal my intestines and live a healthy life was to avoid eating gluten. Food is the only cure.

Imagine being told that you can never eat gluten, in any form, ever again. After months, or even years, of mysterious maladies, you feel grateful to finally have an end to the pain. But for the rest of your life—no gluten.

No more bread. No more beer. No more baked goods. Visit Italy, pass on the pasta. Go to Paris and watch others savor a *pain au chocolat* while you sip coffee. Skip those Sunday morning cinnamon rolls. You cannot eat chocolate chip cookies from your favorite bakery. You cannot grab a slice of pizza from Sal and Carmine's. You cannot even enjoy a bowl of oatmeal in the morning. You cannot have any of it, because it will make you terribly ill.

Your life depends upon it.

Gluten is the glue that holds together baked goods and pasta. In fact, the word *gluten* comes from the same Latin root as "glue." Think of gluten as the glue of wheat, rye, and barley. Its elasticity is why French bread holds together, why angel food cakes rise so high, and why H & H bagels in New York are so wonderfully doughy. When you are diagnosed with celiac disease, you must give up every one of those sensory experiences.

Living gluten-free, however, is not as easy as avoiding bread, beer, and baked goods. Gluten hides insidiously in nearly every processed food, from some commercial ice creams to a few soy milks. Gluten lurks in places one would never suspect. Giving up gluten would be infinitely easier if it just meant never having a pastrami sandwich on rye. However, some slices of pastrami are as likely to make me as sick as the rye bread. Why? Gluten is hidden in thousands of products, in places one would never think to look. Mass-processed meats are often made with gluten to fill out the salami or to make the turkey seem plumper. I would never have guessed that prepackaged meat had wheat in it. Some Popsicles have gluten in them. Homemade Popsicles end up fairly thin because they are just frozen juice. Think about the flour paste most of us made in elementary school. Remember how thick and viscous it grew as you stirred it? Now, imagine that in Popsicles. Most commercial Popsicles, and a hundred other packaged foods, contain gluten. Ketchup can have gluten in it. Soy sauce, light sour cream, and root beer all contain gluten.

Of course, almost no packaged food says: CONTAINS GLUTEN. Gluten can be disguised in the form of modified food starch, hydrolized vegetable protein, malt, dextrins, and even "natural flavors." Corn chips that are fried in the same oil as gluten products can make me sick. Anything packaged that comes in individual pieces—candy, frozen foods, corn tortillas, french fries, or even cashews—could be dusted in flour just before being stuffed in the package. Why? We like everything to look pretty. We cannot have two pieces of chocolate sticking together. I once suffered for two days because of the infinitesimal amount of wheat flour that had been dusted on two chocolate-covered espresso beans.

In order to stay well, those millions who must eat gluten-free have to read every box, decipher every ingredient, and ponder every bite they eat. Restaurants can be a minefield because of hidden flours and cross-contamination. If a food worker forgets to wash his or her hands after dipping something in flour and then prepares a salad, we grow sick. Some people with celiac disease have not eaten in a restaurant in fifteen years. Some subsist on foods in boxes stamped GLUTEN-FREE, switching the prepackaged allegiances of their youth to different packages.

However, with the suffocating tastes of my childhood still on my tongue, I knew that I could not live my food life longing for my old way of eating. Going without packaged food does not mean that life closes down. Instead, the world can bloom open.

Without my familiar meals, I had to seek out other foods that were naturally gluten-free, which I could eat without fear of growing sick. There were dreadful experiments and kitchen disasters: lumpy bread with an underlying whiff of beans; sour pastries that wilted at the touch; funky cookies that spread like bad news through a small town. At sixteen, I gave up experimenting after two weeks of bad veggie burgers. This time, I persisted. I found a quote from my childhood favorite, Julia Child, and stuck it to my refrigerator: "The only stumbling block is the fear of failure. In cooking you've got to have a what-the-hell attitude." I started experimenting with food and trusting those taste buds I had acquired over the years.

Fairly quickly, I realized that I didn't want to find merely adequate substitutions for the foods I was missing, perpetually mourning the fact that they didn't taste like the original. Instead of feeling angry or disappointed that I could never eat a bagel in New York again, I felt elated. The relief was enormous. Finally, I knew the answer.

The answer was *yes*.

I started saying yes to foods I had never eaten before, as long as they did not contain gluten.

Buoyant with energy after years of being flattened from exhaustion, I spent more and more time in the kitchen, teaching myself to cook with whole foods instead of using prepackaged foodstuffs. Soon, I started making my own corn tortillas—much more satisfying than anything I had ever bought in a store—and topping them with chunks of creamy avocado, grated artisanal cheese with spices from Madagascar, and small cherry tomatoes at the height of their season. Soon, I made my own salsa, explosive with peppers and rich with tomato flavor. Polenta appeared on my table at least once a week, and then more often. I let it rest overnight, then grilled thick wedges of it in a fruity olive oil from Spain, and ladled over it a slow-simmered pasta sauce with ten cloves of garlic, a few shavings of nutmeg, and a touch of ginger.

I did not miss gluten.

With all these tastes dancing on my tongue, I wanted more. I bought my food directly from the farmers at Seattle's seasonal markets. I learned how to make jam from the wild blackberries growing by the side of the road in summer. Stocks from scratch, flourless chocolate tortes, or homemade potato chips—nothing daunted me anymore. I started haunting kitchen supply stores, coveting cast-iron cookware and new baking sheets. I talked to farmers and commercial fishermen and chefs who made everything from scratch. I played with my food, in all its sensory pleasures, and then I began to share it with other people. I stopped looking for men to date and instead opened my senses to people who could feed me.

Spurred on by my love of writing and teaching others what I had learned, I started a food Web site called Gluten-Free Girl. I thought that only my fifty-six friends were reading it, but people started coming by my site to read, in hungry droves. Within a few months, I had a loyal readership for my food photographs and recipes. For months on end, in accordance with my own expanding taste, and for the sake of the readers coming back to my Web site, I created recipes spontaneously, such as roasted-pepper risotto, guacamole with cumin and pomegranate seeds, or hummus with kalamata olives and fresh basil. My marinade for salmon made of toasted sesame oil, tamari sauce, and champagne vinegar held a complexity of flavors in one bite.

Going gluten-free invited me to throw open my windows and let the world into my kitchen.

Six months after my diagnosis, I invited my parents over for dinner. We ate a lavish, three-course meal, food my mother would have rejected out of hand when we were younger. To start, I served crunchy crackers made from toasted quinoa, along with a triple-cream cheese, made by an all-women's cheese-making collective in northern California. The main course was an organic chicken from Oregon, roasted with fresh rosemary and Meyer lemons, accompanied by braised fennel and baby bok choy. On the side was a salad of wild greens, local goat cheese, pomegranate seeds, and a light sprinkling of toasted millet. For dessert, we ate a flourless chocolate torte made from Dutch-processed chocolate and Irish butter, studded with fresh raspberries.

My mother marveled at the spread and the smells filling the tiny apartment kitchen. "You made all this for us?" she exclaimed. With every bite, she and my father smiled and sighed, celebrating the tastes. After a few bites of the salad—no croutons from a box, the shallot vinaigrette not poured from a bottle—she looked up at me, tears in her eyes, and said, "This is the best salad I have ever eaten."

That's when I knew I was home. I had finally found food that would fill me, without making me sick, food that anyone could love, even my mother.

3

the ten noble tastes

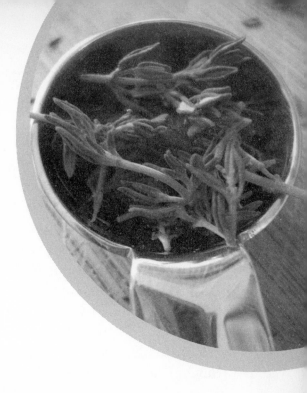

After I found out that I must eat gluten-free, memories of my time in London began drifting back.

For six months, at the end of the twentieth century, I lived in London with a ridiculously wealthy family. How did I end up there? I cannot tell you. I don't mean to be coy. I mean that literally. The confidentiality agreement I signed with them precludes me from telling you any details.

I can share this.

Big bowls of bouillabaisse, with fist-size pieces of lobster dotting the surface of the briny broth. Blue cheese soufflés. Wild mushroom tarts. Fresh melon wrapped in prosciutto. Salty caviar on tiny toasts, caviar flown in from Russia that morning. Fresh-squeezed orange juice in gold-rimmed glasses.

For snacks, the cook arrived at the desk brandishing trays of broiled figs. They tasted decadent, like gourmet candy and expensive restaurants at the same time. She smeared little dabs of the finest French brie on the figs, then put them under the broiler. Five minutes later, and I was sighing with pleasure as I ate. Softly sweet, with a crunch of seeds, everything melting into one, the smooth taste of cheese spreading into the sweetness, and all of it over in thirty seconds. But the taste lingered and fingered its way down to my stomach.

The only aspect of that time that feels warm and clear—like onions and garlic simmering in olive oil—is the food. I had been the girl who ate grilled cheese sandwiches, bags of potato chips, and frozen pizzas all day long. There, I became the woman who tasted truffle oil for the first time and ate enough risotto to make it wonderfully mundane. During my time with the wealthy family, I was exposed to the world of real food, and I wanted more.

One of the best perks of living with this family in London was the chance to visit different cities in Europe at will. Every other weekend, at least, I hopped on a plane to Florence or rode the Chunnel train to Paris. Whether the destination was Amsterdam, Prague, or Dublin, I went on whims and walked by myself through the beautiful streets. Each weekend, I reveled in the chance to be alone in a country where I only knew the food terms. I ate *pain au chocolat* at a boulangerie in Paris just off the Jardin du Luxembourg. I savored the creamy residue of pistachio gelato on my lips, as I sat just off the Piazza di Santa Croce in Florence. I drank twenty-five-cent beers in Prague. I ate so many potatoes in Ireland that I felt fully Irish myself. After all the cloistered claustrophobia of my childhood, I was exultant, just walking down the street by myself, eating a crepe I had bought off a stand on the Champs-Élysées.

One rainy weekend, in Florence, I wandered the city without being able to speak the language at all. I walked up all 422 steps of the Duomo. I stood in front of Michelangelo's *David* by myself, since there were no tourist crowds. I walked along the Arno and thought about my strange life and how I had come to be there. I could feel my mind growing full, deeply sated at these experiences, and nearly ready to stop devouring so hungrily. Later that evening, I stood at the edge of the Piazza della Signoria, an enormous square next to the Uffizi art gallery. On one side loomed epic-size statues of Zeus and David, replicas of the originals still entrancing in their immensity. As I started to walk across the square, rain began falling, hard. People ran, trying to evade the eternal wet. But I had lived near Seattle. Rain didn't scare me. Neither did that impending thunder, rolling across the sky. This is how I came to be the only person in the Piazza della Signoria, with Zeus towering over me, in the middle of a raging lightning storm.

In the end, even I was too wet to stand in the puddles, so I ducked into the nearest restaurant. I entered because of the smells. The aromas of roasted garlic, braised meats, smoked tomatoes, and the sharp snap of pepper lured me in like a lover. A sultry Italian man came to my table and asked me what I wanted. I didn't understand him. We spoke in hand gestures, in futility, until I spread out my hands, palms up, as though to say, "I give up. Bring me what you want." And so he did. He brought an enormous platter of antipasti: beautiful little curlicues of salami and Parma ham, fried goat cheese, glistening pearl onions. But the taste I remember most clearly is the smoked mozzarella. I could tell from the taste that it had just been made, that day, even though I had never tasted fresh mozzarella before. It still smelled warm, as though it had come from the hands that had created it. Creamy, milky, with a certain corresponding sweetness, it was decadent dreamy dumbfounding beauty on the tongue. Slinking across the top was a gorgeous smoky taste, like a wood fire on a cold, wet night, the snap of the fire enough to keep us awake, the gray smoke rising into the sky. I tasted all of this in that cheese.

That's when I knew true richness. It wasn't the luxury to throw away money on parties that impressed, temporarily. It was the taste of that food, made fresh by human hands, with incredible tenderness and pride. That was all I needed.

Everyone should have good food. I don't mean caviar and champagne. Too much of that stuff will leave you feeling glutted and guilty. Instead, after I went gluten-free, I began searching out singular tastes. After cooking every night for a couple of months, I realized that the key to great eating is not secret recipes or training at a culinary school. *It's the ingredients we choose.*

In those years before my celiac diagnosis, food often languished in the refrigerator. I'd plan elaborately for a big meal and then be too physically exhausted to cook for days. Vegetables would shrink into themselves in the crisper drawer. The corners of cheese would start to crack from dryness. Leftovers would wither into some strange concoction that would make me turn my head and wince when I threw it out. I wasted food, and I always felt guilty.

Not anymore.

Those months in London rubbed off on me without my knowing it. After going gluten-free, I adopted the European village method of shopping. Daily jaunts to my favorite little stores sustain me and teach me about great food. I have a friendly relationship with the people who run these places. From asking and listening, I have learned how to choose the freshest foods.

A couple months after I realized I had to eat gluten-free, I began going to a different food store every day. Some people venture to movie theaters or buy CDs for fun. I go to grocery stores. Seattle is suffused with great food emporiums, stocked with sea salts, twenty different vinegars, and cheeses from around the world. Instead of grabbing the cheapest foods I could find, I decided to spend my "fun" money every month on new foods. I explored. I tasted samples. I asked questions. I felt blessed when I started exploring the Pike Place Market, a nearly one-hundred-year-old farmers' market on the water, with dozens of little stalls and shops. I bought my meats at Don and Joe's, the stall at the front of the Market, where the butchers have calloused hands and friendly faces. I sampled great cheeses at DeLaurenti's. I found pomegranate molasses at the Souk, the tiny sliver of a store that sold Middle Eastern food.

One day, I wandered into a warehouse and found my idea of heaven. Chef Shop, which is predominantly an online source for gourmet foods from around the world, happens to be physically situated in Seattle. When I first walked in, I meant to stay for ten or fifteen minutes. Instead, I had to call the friend I was meeting for coffee and tell her I would meet her the next day. Tall shelves extending to the ceiling contained bottles of olive oil, jars of honey, packages of beans, and bars of chocolate. I walked in a daze, for a moment, until an employee interrupted my reverie with the offer of an olive oil tasting. Strange, I thought. But why not?

He poured a drop of greenish oil on a white plastic spoon and extended it toward me. I sipped and tipped my head back to taste it fully. It sang of summer. I tried another, which was as mellow as butter. The third one tasted just like grass, distilled. I looked at the man offering me these gifts with a puzzled look. "How do they taste so different?" I asked him. He laughed and told me a little about the way olive oils are produced, how the land the olives are grown on makes a difference in the taste. We hadn't even started sampling the flavored olive oils yet. (Later, a black truffle oil from a farmer in Umbria made me decide on the spot to visit Umbria some day, just so I could meet that farmer.) Soon, I was clutching a Meyer lemon olive oil from northern California in my hands. Noble sour vinegar, Le Puy lentils from France, spice rubs from Morocco, and dried chiles from Mexico—the choices made me feel a little dizzy. But I wanted more.

The folks at Chef Shop quickly became friends. I stopped in nearly every week, eager to see what they had in store for me. The owners, Tim and Eliza, search the world for exquisite ingredients for people looking to make restaurant-quality food at home. Over time, by sampling different oils and vinegars and making meals with them, I learned that a real cook insists on the best ingredients.

Once I realized what a difference an exquisite olive oil could make, I was determined to buy the best of every food. The guys at my favorite produce stand at the Market—Sosio's produce, where every person is friendly flirtatious—introduced me to eating foods in season: fava beans, orange cauliflower, and the joys of the first strawberry of spring. Even though I love grocery stores, I could never discover as much in small bites if I made a list and bought all my food for the week in one shopping trip.

Everyone deserves good food. Not just the wealthy or famous. Everyone. With that in mind, here is my guide to the ten foods I have learned to splurge on after going gluten-free, the foods that make all my meals. With just a bit of money and mindfulness, you can live richly.

1. high-quality oils

When I was in the fifth grade, my parents owned a neon green VW Rabbit, a cramped and ludicrous car. That car broke down, often. My teacher parents could not afford the constant trips to the mechanic. When the pillbug of a car refused to start one more time, my father decided to take it on. He taught literature and film history. He knew nothing about cars. Our next-door neighbor, Mike, knew a little about cars, after being alive for ninety years. This unlikely pair was huddled over the engine, in front of our yard. After an hour of tinkering, they still had not managed to make the engine turn over.

My mother, always with an answer, strode out to the car and stood beside them. "It sounds like it needs an oiling. It needs some WD-40," she said. My father and Mike both disdained her, insisting it could not be that. My mother went back into the house. However, my mother rarely allowed herself to be silenced, and she certainly didn't like being treated like the little woman. She came marching back out of the house, this time clutching a jug of vegetable oil.

You remember that vegetable oil. Mrs. Brady said you should cook with its goodness, for fine American foods. I remember the image of a pile of fried chicken on a plate, sunshine spilling in the windows through the checkered curtains. This vegetable oil, however, was pretty cheap. It was a blend of oils—soy, safflower, and corn—with a slightly different blend every time, depending on what was cheapest at the market at the time it was bottled. At that point in my life, I had never even heard of olive oil. As my father recently said to me, "That would have only been available in the 'ethnic' markets, and we didn't shop there."

However, my father often told the story of a dinner he ate one night, at an Italian restaurant thirty miles from home. He and my mother ate there just after they had started dating, on the recommendation of a friend of his family. Rather than prepackaged foods and boil-in-a-bag meals, this restaurant served antipasti, salads, fresh pasta, and all that is authentic Italian food. My father used to tell my brother and me, in the most lavish details, about every bite of the seven courses they ate. Of course, when I was a kid, I thought, "Why don't you stop telling me about this and take me there?" Now I wonder if he wasn't just amazed at the olive oil they must have used.

No, in our house, we only had vegetable oil, the oil so light it looked almost like water. The oil was sold in enormous jugs, like the jug my mother was carrying in her clenched hand toward the VW Rabbit.

She strode toward the men, who were bent over the car and lost in serious conversation about the alternator and the timing belt. They didn't notice my mother at first. When they did see her coming toward them with the jug of oil, they stood in front of the engine, their mouths open, not moving. They saw—they couldn't stop her.

My mother walked right up to the open hood of the car, opened the cap on that plastic jug, and poured a big glug of the oil on the dusty engine. And then she insisted that my incredulous father get in the car, turn the key, and try to start it. He scoffed and grew angry, but he did what he was told.

The car started.

Do you really want to cook with oil like that?

Cooking with quality oils truly makes a difference in the taste of food. These days, extra virgin olive oil is fairly ubiquitous in supermarkets. We have made great food strides in this country. However, after I discovered the taste of olive oil in my twenties, I thought I was really being a gourmet by buying an eight-dollar bottle from the supermarket, instead of spending two dollars on a jug of vegetable oil. It took me years to realize that spending twenty-five dollars on a bottle of truly outstanding olive oil is worth it, sometimes.

One day last year, I slurped a spoonful of olive oil from Sicily at Chef Shop without any accompaniment. It tasted like sharp green olives, warmed by the sun. I closed my eyes to experience it more fully. When I looked at the price tag, I hesitated for a moment. But I had to follow that taste. At home, I made homemade pesto, with organic basil and toasted pine nuts, with olive oil slowly drizzled in. That bright-green taste melded all the flavors together. I went to bed happy that night.

All olive oils are not the same. Some varieties are described as tasting green—you can almost taste the grass beneath the olive trees. Others are fruity and offer fullness to the mouth. Some oils have such a peppery bite at the back of the tongue that you might think they were spiked. But all great olive oils taste alive. They have a true taste, like different varieties of wine. I usually have several bottles in my home at one time now.

I made the mistake, when I first started buying good olive oil, of making everything with that twenty-five-dollar bottle of olive oil. That bottle emptied out alarmingly fast. Someone who truly knows food taught me instead to combine oils for different methods of cooking. Now I fill an empty cruet one-quarter full with my favorite olive oil and then fill it the rest of the way with a high-quality canola or safflower oil. That way, I get a bit of that olive oil taste in my seared fish, but I don't use the entire bottle. Most dishes require a more neutral taste, besides. Use great olive oil in dishes where its taste truly matters: concocting salad dressings; finishing off sauces; drizzling over soup; lavishing on good, gluten-free bread; or finishing a risotto. When the taste of the olive oil shines through, that's the time to bring out the twenty-five-dollar bottle.

After my olive oil discoveries, I branched out into other oils as well. I have become a big fan of walnut oil, particularly one made by a family in France that does not toast the walnuts before pressing them. A thin stream of that oil tastes like condensed walnuts, with no other taste muddling the senses. Sesame oil seems essential for any kind of Asian foods, as it complements those flavors especially well. I've come to love a few drops of chili oil in Thai stir-fries and Vietnamese soups as well. Pumpkin seed oil, which is normally dark and quite thick, enlivens my baby bok choy in the middle of the winter. And truffle oil, although it can be quite expensive, can make a profound difference in food. A few drops on the top of a mushroom risotto brings out the decadent flavors even more fully.

The description of all these oils may make you feel as though you need to spend an entire month's paycheck lining your pantry shelves in order to cook well. Think about how expensive fast food and junk food truly is. Splurging on high-quality oils is a much better choice.

2. salts

My father always salts his food, before he even tastes it. To this day, no matter what plate is put in front of him, he eyes the food, then reaches for the saltshaker. Usually, he showers the food with salt, until it looks like dandruff on his dinner.

"Dad!" I usually say. "You haven't even tasted it yet!"

He shrugs, then says to me, "I can just tell from looking at the food. It needed more salt."

This makes sense only if you think about how salty packaged food is. The sodium content of most TV dinners is enough to make an elephant feel bloated. Every potato chip tastes as though you are eating a salt lick. Packaged pasta dinners, hot dogs, and even luncheon meats—it feels as though the first ingredient really should be listed as salt.

Once I stepped away from the terrible tastes of my childhood, I learned I could have more tastes on my tongue than salt. Once I started cooking my own food from scratch, I learned to truly season my food. Once I bought good salts, my food started tasting like itself.

It always used to confuse me when I read recipes that listed salt at the last moment, with the almost flippant instructions to "season to taste." What did that mean? I thought—and I know I'm not alone—that it meant I should put enough salt into the food to make it taste salty. Now I know differently. Cooking is a physical process, of the body, not of the mind. No one should serve food before tasting it. Once you have been cooking for a while, you will develop a sense of whether that soup needs a pinch of salt or a teaspoon. But still, we need to taste our food as we make it. Many a time, I have made a pot of soup and it tasted fine. A little flat, perhaps, but perfectly decent. Before I started devoting myself to food, I would have served that soup to everyone at the table, then watched them all reach for the saltshaker, like my father. But now, when the soup tastes a little flat, I know it needs a bit more salt. I pinch in a bit of salt, crunching it between my fingers, and then I stir the soup. Suddenly, the soup tastes vibrant, singing through the singular tastes to create a harmony of flavors, something beyond itself. The salt doesn't make it salty. The salt simply allows the soup to come alive.

I never use a saltshaker anymore. I like the physical sensation of pinching the salt between my fingers. This is why I keep a little dish of kosher salt on the top of the stove. I have learned to hold my fingers high above my food, about chest-level, when I am seasoning. This distributes the salt evenly in the food. Before going gluten-free, I tossed salt into a pan from an inch above the surface of the food. That often made the food too salty for other people.

Well, except for my father, of course.

Once you have learned to season your food by trial and error, you might be wondering, which salt should I use? When I was a kid, we only had one salt: the big blue container of table salt, with the girl under the umbrella, pouring salt on the sidewalk to show that it would still pour. Well, unfortunately, the only reason this happens is that most table salt is threaded through with anticaking agents. In other words, there is more than salt in your salt.

Every chef I know uses kosher salt, whether for braising meats or for making soups. Kosher salt is light and slightly larger than table salt. It has a flakiness to it that makes it spread through the food more easily than heavier sea salt can. The most common brand of kosher salt also comes with anticaking agents, so the natural flavor of the salt is rather masked. I'm a big fan of Diamond Crystal kosher salt. One small taste on the tongue and everything starts to wake up. Kosher salt is much smaller than sea salt, which makes it easier to splash into the food.

Sea salt. Oh my, this could take a while. Celtic sea salt, orange lava sea salt from Hawaii, truffle sea salt, fennel sea salt, black volcanic sea salt—these are starting to seem like designer labels. In essence, sea salt is harvested from seawater, stored in traps, then left to evaporate in the sun. Salt that comes from this process is much coarser than table salt or kosher salt. It has a slight humidity to it and tastes faintly of the sea. Most sea salt is harvested in France, although one of my favorites comes from off the coast of the United Kingdom. *Fleur de sel*, the top layer of that harvest, is clean and white and light. This is the most commonly available sea salt. *Sel gris* is fairly gray, much denser, and moister than *fleur de sel.* I use this only sparingly, when I really want my food to be reminiscent of the ocean.

Sea salt, I have discovered the hard way, works best when you brandish it at the last moment, sprinkling it on the top of food just before serving it. Take my word for it—you don't want to use coarse sea salt in your baked goods. Not unless you want your gluten-free gingerbread to contain lumps of salt that will make your family wince.

As with all these ingredients, I recommend going to a good kitchen store or a gourmet-food store and sampling. Take a small nibble of Maldon sea salt and crunch its huge, pyramid-shaped flakes between your fingers, then let the crystals shower down upon your food. I adore the lightness of this salt, and right now, it's the one I use most often. Strange as this may sound, it's the saltiest of the salts out there. I'm also fond of an herbed sea salt called Vignalta, which is produced in Venice, Italy. Harvested in the late summer, the salt is also pounded with rosemary, sage, garlic, and pepper. Whenever someone comes to my house for dinner, I ask her to put her nose in the jar of this salt. She always comes up smiling. If I want to feel decadent on a weekday afternoon, I season my fresh-popped corn with a pinch of truffle salt.

3. vinegars

When I was a kid, we ate salads nearly every night. We had iceberg lettuce—white and seemingly devoid of any nutrition—one-quarter of a pale tomato, and a glurb of bottled salad dressing. One night we had blue cheese dressing from a bottle, and then the next we had a viscous "Italian" dressing. They had nearly the same texture, because they were poured from bottles and packed with preservatives.

Once in a while, however, my parents bought takeout from a Mexican restaurant a few miles from our home. It was in the "bad" part of town, I remember, so I could never go with my father when he went to pick up the food.

I don't remember any of the other food. The reason I don't remember the other food is that their salads were so damned good.

The lettuce was dark green, not icy white like our iceberg. On top of the lettuce was shredded Monterey Jack cheese. In our house, the cheese arrived already grated, in a bag. That made the eating months away from the grating, which left the cheese stale and stiff. But the cheese from this restaurant lay in soft tendrils on the bed of green lettuce, waiting for the dressing.

The dressing was tart and puckery—my mouth always bunched around each bite after I took it in. The oil base beneath it was rich and slithery, like nothing I had ever experienced. And there were layers of taste after the vivid sharpness of the first bite. It tasted like the first rush of an airplane ride, when the wheels lift off the ground. That salad dressing made me think of clear, thin air, high atop mountains. I had visions of eating somewhere far away, the hot sun nudging the small circle of shade in which I sat.

I'm not certain of the exact ingredients in that salad dressing. But as an adult, when I first tasted good red wine vinegar, I knew. That's what they did. They used olive oil and red wine vinegar, heavy on the vinegar.

In my childhood home—and most houses in the United States at the time—there was only one kind of vinegar: white vinegar. Acrid and clear, it doubled as the second ingredient in salad dressings my mother made on special occasions and as an all-purpose cleaner. Some people clean their windows by dousing newspapers in white vinegar and making vigorous circles on the glass. Others use it as a stain remover on carpets. I remember my mother pouring it through the coffeemaker once a week to clean the appliance of the grounds and gunk, which left the house smelling foul.

I'm supposed to eat this stuff?

Now a dozen different vinegars stand on my kitchen shelves, each of them lending a different taste to the foods I eat. I splash good rice wine vinegar into boiling water to make perfect poached eggs. Champagne vinegar flavors my daily salad dressing, which I whip up in the blender once a week; I then pour its delicate tartness onto wild greens, goat cheese, and pumpkin seeds. I have made a reduction sauce from my favorite balsamic vinegar, flavored with fig, to pour over roast pork loin and butternut squash. In the summer, I splash a tomato vinegar—amber like bottled sunshine—from Austria over heirloom tomatoes, let them marinate, then throw them into gluten-free pasta salads for a taste experience that takes people to places they never expected.

Experiment and play. Find vinegars that work for you. Then buy another bottle.

4. cheeses

Until I was in my late twenties, I thought that Parmesan cheese meant one thing: clumped, sawdust-dry, and shaken from a big green can. We all ate that so-called Parmesan cheese. Was it even cheese? I've never been sure. It could have been reconstituted cheese product, for all I know. It doesn't taste anything like the real Parmigiano-Reggiano. I'm sure that green can was full of gluten. But that's what I ate, when my parents had "Italian" dinners: spaghetti with giant meatballs, sauce poured from a jar into a saucepan, then a fast shake from the green can. Do you know that no matter how hot that sauce was, the cheese never melted? It just stayed there, sagging on top of the spaghetti.

The cheese I ate when I was a kid is vile to me now. Enormous logs of semisoft, dyed orange substance, vaguely tasting of cheddar, but mostly just tasting pasty. It didn't melt on the tongue. Instead, it stayed filmy on my teeth for hours. Cheese spread was a salty, day-glow orange cheese product, thick enough to stay one consistency in a little glass jar. I remember the port wine flavor most because it felt like luxury to me when I was a kid. There was also the cheese spread with bacon bits suspended in the midst of it. Sometimes I flipped open the little metal lid, stuck my finger in the cheese spread, and watched game shows while I ate the entire jar. Each slice of American cheese was wrapped in clear plastic, and the stack was swathed in another layer of thick plastic. And the taste? I cannot describe the taste. I don't think it had a taste.

Junk food has one taste. A handful of cheesy puffs always tastes the same: salty, with a chemical cheese taste and a styrofoam consistency. Open any bag, anywhere in the world, and they will always taste the same.

But take one bite of a truly great cheese, close your eyes, and be astonished by the layers of subtlety. I will never forget the first time I tasted Gouda. When I was sixteen, my father was given a Fulbright scholarship to teach at a polytechnic institute in London, which meant my family exchanged houses, cars, and lives with a British family. The food we encountered there sometimes horrified me, but we found much better cheeses in Great Britain than we ever had in Los Angeles.

Sitting in the living room of our London house, pale sunlight filtering through the windows, I took a bite of the soft cheese from Holland. First, I tasted milkiness, like a bucket of warm milk condensed into one bite. It was chewy, with a true texture, which forced my teeth to bite down. After a moment, there was a hint of something almost smoky at the back of my mouth. My tongue noticed the nubbly texture where the cheese met the waxy red rind. And in the end, it all smelled clean, like pastures in spring.

My dear friend Françoise has taught me the French way of being with cheese. Have only the best. Have only a small amount. When food tastes truly, truly great, I don't need more than a few mouthfuls to be sated.

Now I am a cheese fiend. Every week, I try something new. Provolone, Mahon, Fontina, Asiago—I will eat them all, and happily. Twenty years ago, I didn't know they existed. I have come to depend on soft chèvre, spread on quinoa crackers or dropped on top of a salad of wild greens. I eat some nearly every day. When I was a kid, I did not even know that goats made milk, much less the subtle cheese that comes from it. I know I'm not the only one. Recently, I was in a chain grocery store, stranded in a part of Seattle I didn't know. Planning ahead for a picnic, I asked one of the checkers if they had any goat cheese. She scrunched up her face at me, seemingly in disgust. "I've never heard of that. People eat that?" I tried to convince her that yes, we do. She didn't look convinced. She has no idea what she is missing.

One word of caution, sadly, for those of you reading who cannot eat gluten: we have to avoid the blue cheeses. Maybe. All the best blue cheeses—such as Roquefort, Gorgonzola, and Stilton—are threaded through with a thin line of mold. That mold was, for the most part, started from bread, and then injected into the cheese as it aged. In fact, legend has it that the first Roquefort cheese came into existence because a shepherdess in the south of France accidentally left her cheese-on-rye sandwich in a cave near Roquefort-sur-Soulzon. When she returned a few weeks later, she found penicillin mold lining the walls of the cave. How she decided to put that into cheese is anyone's guess, but that is reputed to be the birth of blue cheese. Since cheesemakers like to keep their process secret, it's not entirely clear which blue cheeses are started from bread molds and which are not. It's best to ask each individual cheese maker. Me? Unfortunately, I have decided to simply stay away from them, after several gluten reactions.

But that's okay. There are plenty of other cheeses to savor.

5. fresh herbs

Remember that terrible Parmesan cheese from a can that topped our spaghetti? It was accompanied by one herb flavoring called "Italian seasoning." Shaken from a plastic container, this popular spice showed up in any foods my mother made that were supposed to be gourmet. Sometimes she patted the gray-green flakes into soft butter, then spread it on French bread from the grocery store and baked it in the oven, covered in tin foil. Or she might douse the top of the pizza that arrived at the door in the hands of a teenage delivery guy, just to make it more "authentic." I never had any idea what was in Italian seasoning. In fact, until I was well into my twenties, I honestly thought all foods in Italy were made by shaking some of this magic stuff from a jar.

Now I know better, after having eaten in Italy and learning how to cook well. Looking at the label of that seasoning, I see that it contains basil, marjoram, oregano, rosemary, sage, savory, and thyme. How much better would our foods have been if we had learned to cook with those herbs, fresh?

And I don't even want to talk about the fact that we used garlic powder from a jar instead of fresh garlic cloves.

There simply is no substitute for fresh herbs. I learned that, happily, once I scooted back in the kitchen after my celiac diagnosis. Again, I am blessed to live in Seattle, where the farmers' markets on the weekend offer a profusion of fresh herbs. When the farmers' markets are not open in the winter, there are still small packages of fresh herbs available in stores, and most of them are organic. They might seem terribly expensive at first—why spend three dollars on a tiny package of fresh basil when I can buy an entire bottle of dried basil for that much?—but fresh herbs are worth the expense.

At first, I was delighted to experiment with herbs whose names were familiar. Fresh rosemary has a smell unlike anything else: pungent, sharp, a bit like pine trees, enormously kind. I learned from watching chef Jamie Oliver on television how to dip the needles into boiling water before I put them in my roast chicken, so the essential oils release themselves more readily. Take one whiff of rosemary that way and you are likely to fall over.

One of the reasons I always hesitated to buy so many fresh herbs is that they seemed to go bad and black very quickly. However, that happened because I was not storing them correctly. Now I buy fresh herbs in small doses, only when I need them. If I have any left over, I wrap it with a wet paper towel and put it in a resealable bag. Every day after that, I use a little more, throwing away what is starting to wither and dry out. I also save all the woody stems of certain herbs—such as thyme, marjoram, and rosemary—in a bowl on top of my kitchen shelves, for the stocks I make every Sunday. Those stems give my homemade stock an incredible depth that no can or box of stock can ever touch.

6. unfamiliar flavors

When I lived in London as a teenager, I was astonished to find that my diet at home tasted wildly varied in comparison to the English way of eating. Everything there was fried, breaded, and tasted of meat. Foods came with weird names—toad in the hole, bubble and squeak, and spotted dick—but they all tasted of sausages, suet, and sweets. The rest of the world had not truly entered the United Kingdom yet, excluding the corner Tandoori takeaways, and people were still cooking with the legacy of the Blitz in mind. Translation: my goodness, everything tasted bland. I never once ate garlic the entire year I lived there.

Oh sure, I had eaten that transcendent piece of Gouda. Dairy—especially cream and butter—was better in London than it had been at home. But when I lived in Great Britain the year I was sixteen, the single spice used in the kitchens we visited was salt. (Thank goodness, everything has changed since then.)

Our taste buds were so dulled from eating in London that our family once made a raid on the food department at Harrods. We ran through the aisles searching out all the American food we could find. Triumphant, we went back to our crummy little Fiat with bags filled with Mexican-style frozen dinners from Texas, big bags of Fritos, and a box of Lucky Charms. My father drove for a bit toward home, and then we couldn't stand it. We had to eat some. That's how we came to be parked in front of Charles Dickens's childhood home, eating an entire jar of dill pickle chips.

That was our version of an expansion of tastes.

There is no avoiding the fact that most Americans eat within a narrow range of tastes. But there is an entire world of extraordinary flavors out there—faintly sweet; smells-of-the-sea salty; pucker-up-the-lips bitter; kick-in-the-stomach sour; make-me-moan umami—and life simply grows more exciting with each exposure to a wider variety of tastes in the mouth.

When I went gluten-free, and thus spent as much time in my kitchen as I could, I started experimenting with tastes, enjoying the playing of flavors, savoring what resonated, and throwing out the rest. Along the way, I discovered some spices from around the world that I had never heard of, much less cooked with, before I let the world into my kitchen.

The faint memory of that dash of red atop deviled eggs led me to play with paprika, also known as Hungarian paprika. It is fine, sweet, and mild. But then I found smoked paprika. Smoked paprika comes from Spain, where farmers smoke several different peppers in layers of oakwood for weeks. After they are smoked and dried, the peppers are ground into paprika.

One whiff convinced me. Dusky red, the spice smells deeply of wood-fire smoke, the kind where everyone relaxes and tells stories as they look into the flames. It bites at the nose, playfully, inviting another sniff. I started cooking with it.

A few months later, pomegranate molasses started creeping into my consciousness. My friend Molly mentioned that she had carried a jar back from Manhattan on one of her last jaunts. "Hmm," I thought, "if it's that special, why am I not cooking with it?" I started noticing it in recipes in my favorite cooking magazines. What did they know that I didn't? And finally, when I was laid up on the couch with a badly sprained ankle, my friend Dorothy brought me a little jar of the elixir.

I dipped my little finger into the dark liquid and sipped from its tip. A wave of that tangy, assertive sweetness that comes from pomegranate seeds, followed by the dark allure of molasses. Bright and alive, no blandness there. I knew that I had to cook with it.

playing with pomegranate molasses

Just after I began experimenting with food, I had my friends Merida and Eric over for dinner. There were a dozen little dishes, a flurry of appetizers, and me standing flushed and expectant in front of the stove.

When I told Eric I was making chicken thighs with toasted cashews and pistachios, quick braised in lemon zest and pomegranate molasses, he stared at me. But when he took his first bite, he looked up to the sky for a moment and groaned from the gorgeous taste. Immediately, he raised his wineglass. Merida and I did, too. And here's the toast he gave us: "To the night that Shauna is now officially not kidding around."

Chicken Thighs Braised in Pomegranate Molasses

8 tablespoons high-quality olive oil
4 tablespoons unsalted butter
8 chicken thighs, bone in and skin on
1 large white onion, chopped
8 cloves garlic, peeled and chopped
3 cups chicken stock
8 tablespoons pomegranate molasses
juice of 1 lemon
2 tablespoons sugar
1 teaspoon kosher salt
1 teaspoon cracked black pepper
½ cup cashews
½ cup pistachios, raw and unsalted
zest of 1 lemon

Preheating. Preheat the oven to 425 degrees F.

Browning the chicken thighs. Heat 3 tablespoons of the olive oil, along with the butter, in a heavy saucepan or skillet over medium-high heat. When the mixture has become a hot liquid, add the chicken thighs. Brown them quickly, just 1 or 2 minutes on each side. Put them in a roasting pan and set aside.

Sautéing the onion and garlic. Add the remaining oil and the chopped onion to the saucepan and cook until it is soft, about 2 minutes. Then add the garlic and sauté for another 2 minutes.

Making the fragrant mixture. When the onion and garlic are soft and golden, add the chicken stock, pomegranate molasses, and lemon juice. Bring to a boil. Add the sugar. Cook for 1 minute. Add the salt and pepper.

Baking the chicken. Pour the stock and molasses mixture over the chicken thighs. Cover the pan with aluminum foil and put it into the oven. Bake for 45 minutes, or until the chicken is tender and the internal temperature reads 165 degrees F on your meat thermometer.

Toasting the nuts. Ten minutes before the chicken has finished baking, put the nuts in a skillet and place it into the oven alongside the chicken. Toss the nuts a few times while toasting to make sure they do not burn.

Serving the chicken. Remove the chicken and the nuts from the oven. Place the chicken thighs on a platter. Pour the molasses sauce into a saucepan and bring it to a boil over medium-high heat. Let it simmer for about 10 minutes, or until the sauce begins to thicken. Whisk in 1 tablespoon of butter and the lemon zest. Remove from the heat. Pour the sauce over the chicken thighs. Sprinkle on the toasted nuts and serve.

Feeds 4.

There is no end to the new flavors I want to try. I have just started experimenting with sumac, a sour spice common to the Middle

East, where it is used in place of lemons for astringency. I was introduced to fenugreek through Ethiopian cuisine. My friend Sonora gave me tamarind candies from India, and my mind raced with possibilities.

Once I realized that my food choices would be limited by not being able to eat gluten, I opened my mind to the way the rest of the world eats. I am so grateful. I cannot imagine going back to the way I used to taste my food.

7. butter and dairy products

I dreaded the plastic tub in the door of my grandparents' refrigerator. My grandmother, you see, grew up during the Great Depression, and so she hoarded and scraped all her days. This is why we were always cold in that house. Grandma shouted at us if we turned the heater above 63 degrees. If she caught us throwing out an empty can with half a spoonful of sauce still left in it, or if we did not clean our plates as if a dog had licked it, she launched into a tirade about the wastefulness of our generation. My grandmother would not throw out a single margarine wrapper without first scraping off the last bits left on it. She saved every scrumble of balled-up margarine bits and old crumbs in a white margarine tub. Reaching for some margarine for my morning toast, I would open the plastic lid, then scrunch up my face and turn away.

Whenever someone talks about margarine, I think about that tub in my grandmother's refrigerator. Sure, she was saving a few pennies with her scraping and shouting. But what quality of life was she giving herself, and us?

There is simply nothing like real butter. The first taste is smooth and full and has a certain cleanness. Then comes rushing in a hint of richness, as the butter starts to melt around the tongue. High, clear notes sing out. Like good cheese, butter has a taste of its origins—pastures, sunlight, green grass, and a farmer who wakes up early to milk the cows. Give me this taste, any time, over pale-tasting margarine.

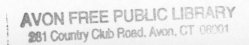

When I was growing up, the popular belief was that butter was evil, because of the dangers of saturated fats and cholesterol. Later, it became clear that the overprocessing required to construct margarine was far worse for our hearts than butter. I am not a medical expert, but I know my own story. I feel better, and I eat less, when I cook with butter. When the real tastes sing out of a dish, clear and excited, I am less inclined to return for seconds when I am not actually hungry. It seems to me now that I ate, and ate more, as a kid, because I was desperately searching for real tastes. When I eat food made with great butter, I savor those tastes more. I slow down.

As with all these other ingredients, I encourage you to experiment and figure out what works for you. I'm fond of a sunny-yellow butter from Ireland, far softer than American butters. On average, most European butters contain more butterfat than American butters, which is what makes them feel so much richer in the mouth.

Salted or unsalted butter? I erroneously believed that salted butter was for cooking and unsalted butter for baked goods. The fact is—and good chefs will back me up on this—unsalted butter is better for both kinds of work. Unsalted butter is fresher (sometimes salt acts as a preservative for mediocre butter far away from its source), has a cleaner taste, and will not overload your food with sodium. With unsalted butter, you can season the food to your taste. The only time I buy salted butter now is when I will use it as a topping for my gluten-free bread. Even then, I only buy a butter from France that has sea salt pounded into it.

The need to buy the finest ingredients continues with other dairy products as well. For a while, I bought a sour cream made in Seattle, because I like to buy local. It seemed wholesome and fresh, even though it didn't taste quite like my ideal conception of sour cream. Then, one day, I read the label more carefully. This sour cream contained nearly a dozen ingredients other than cream: carrageenan, guar gum, xanthan gum, salt, whey, and annatto for coloring. At least the modified starch in the sour cream was corn starch, which made it gluten-free, but why did the makers use any starch to modify the sour cream? For seventy cents more, I bought a sour cream with one ingredient: cream. Do I need to describe the difference in taste? The second one tasted far more full, rich, and inviting.

Most "light" sour creams and cottage cheeses, fat-free cheese, and other atrocities often contain gluten. How else to make a thin, fat-free dairy product taste like the real thing? Pump it full of modified food starch, and then we will all be fooled. By force, I switched to full-fat sour cream and cheeses when I went gluten-free. I have never regretted that turn of events, because my mouth is always happy. So is my body, since eating the best dairy products has satisfied me more deeply than a terrible simulacrum ever could.

Don't let me start on the joys of crème fraîche.

8. chocolate

I have eaten enough bad chocolate to last me several lifetimes—overly sweet milk chocolate filled with nuts or caramels or nougat, stuffed with preservatives and artificial flavors. They were sweet, flat-out sweet, and had one level of taste: sweet. At Halloween every year, I ate so many mini-bars of chocolate and Tootsie Rolls, pulled from my bag when I returned home from a surfeit of door knocking and broad smiling, that I could not tell the difference between the various brands, after a while. They were simply chocolate candy bars. Sweet.

I didn't eat dark chocolate until my late twenties, when I had moved to my little island off Seattle. A friend of mine invited me over for coffee and chocolate after school one day. Ready for instant coffee and drugstore candy bars, I was astonished to find something else waiting for me. We sat around the small table in the kitchen, laughing and talking as early autumn light came through the sliding glass doors. Tita poured me a cup of coffee, dark-roasted black liquid steaming into the air, the smooth, acrid aroma insinuating itself into my nose. I took a sip, and I slipped into a reverie. Just as I was ready to thank her in little trills, she opened up a wrapper and extracted several squares of dark chocolate. The chocolate was melting, slightly, at the touch of her fingers. She held out a square, and it landed in my palm. I lifted it and noticed the trail of melted chocolate left there. Eager to eat it, I placed the chocolate on my tongue, and then I closed my mouth. Solid and liquid at the same time, melting on the corners of my teeth, the chocolate filled my mouth with its sensations. Bright with darkness, no bitter patches, smooth and slowly dissipating. My tongue probed around it, trying to find all the tastes. And there was time, because good chocolate takes long minutes to melt. But soon, too soon, there was only a tiny bit on the tip of my tongue, and then it was gone.

I have never forgotten that first taste of dark chocolate. I have never gone back to bad chocolate after that. I've become a chocolate snob, because I deserve it. And what I have found is that one small square of truly fine chocolate fills the place that once took an entire bag of cheap chocolate. Anything that doesn't taste great when you give it your full attention isn't worth your time.

There are good reasons to buy good chocolate. Chocolate, as you probably know, has some mysterious substances in it that trigger a rush of pheromones in a woman's body, which can mimic the feeling of being in love. More important, scientists have identified that dark chocolate—the only chocolate in my house—has powerful antioxidants. Chocolate, like a glass of red wine, green tea, and even coffee, stimulates the antioxidants in our bodies that fight free radicals, which destroy cells and cause abnormal growths. Even hot chocolate could be helpful. Some doctors are advocating that we eat an ounce of dark chocolate a day.

I can live with that.

There are several wonderful chocolate bars on the market made by companies that take precautions to ensure that gluten does not enter their product. I'm fond of Dagoba chocolates, which are organic, ingeniously flavored (lavender, lime, chai with ginger), and completely gluten-free. During the winter, I drink cup after cup of their hot chocolate, made with chiles and cinnamon, on glowering gray afternoons. Made by a thoughtful company in Ashland, Oregon, dedicated to sustainability and free trade, Dagoba is one of the most exquisite-tasting chocolates in the world. In fact, the *San Francisco Chronicle* voted it the best dark chocolate in the world in 2005.

You see? Gluten-free can certainly be good.

the pastry chef and the gluten-free girl

David Lebovitz—former pastry chef at Chez Panisse, author of gorgeous cookbooks full of spectacular desserts, expert guide of chocolate tours in Paris—gestured toward me in the audience of a cooking class in Seattle. He had been showing his hungry audience how to make spectacular treats. Luckily, most of them didn't require gluten: spiced nuts with fleur de sel; Parisian hot chocolate; and Gâteau Bastille, which involved lots of tiny pieces of prunes, bittersweet chocolate, and heavy cream, but no flour. Before he demonstrated how to make the next decadence, he drew everyone's attention to me, and said, "I'd like to point out the Gluten-Free Girl. Shauna and I met online."

You see, David has a fabulous Web site, dedicated to chocolate, life in Paris, and his sardonic sense of humor. We had been writing back and forth for months, friends before we ever met. Because I was in the audience, David sweetly decided to make chocolate financiers, gluten-free. Instead of the one tablespoon of flour that the recipe called for, he just used another tablespoon of Dutch-processed, unsweetened cocoa powder. And let me tell you, they were fantastic. He told us that in Paris, people eat these tiny little chocolate perfections as a late-afternoon snack. Just a few rich, chocolate bites, with no hint of cloying, tides everyone over until dinner.

That's an afternoon tradition I could sustain.

Chocolate Financiers
(courtesy of David Lebovitz)

6 tablespoons unsalted butter
1 cup almond flour

4 tablespoons Dutch-process unsweetened cocoa powder
⅛ teaspoon salt
¾ cup powdered sugar
⅓ cup egg whites
¼ teaspoon almond extract

Preparing to bake. Preheat the oven to 400 degrees F. Lightly grease and flour financier molds or mini-muffin tins. Melt the butter in a small saucepan and set it aside until it reaches room temperature.

Making the batter. Mix the almond flour with the cocoa powder, salt, and powdered sugar. Stir the egg whites and almond extract into the almond mixture, then gradually stir in the melted butter until incorporated and smooth. Spoon the batter into the molds, filling them three-quarters full.

Baking the financiers. Bake the financiers for 10 to 15 minutes, until the cookies are slightly puffed and springy to the touch. Remove them from the oven and let cool completely before removing the financiers from the molds.

Suggestions. Once cooled, financiers can be kept in an airtight container at room temperature for up to one week.

Makes about 15 one-inch financiers.

9. coffee

When I tell people from other places that I live in Seattle, they always ask me two things: "Doesn't it rain a lot there?" and "So, do you drink a lot of coffee?"

No, not so much. New York City actually has more inches of rain per year than Seattle. Besides, when was the last time you truly listened to the gentle pattering of rain on the roof? If I lived in a place where the rain was sporadic, I'd feel bereft. So it rains, but not as much as the bad press likes to claim.

And coffee? Why, yes. Yes, I do.

Early in the morning, when I stumble into the kitchen at 6:02 A.M., the blat of the alarm clock still ringing in my ears, I'm only thinking of one action: flipping the switch of the coffeepot. The night before, I filled it with water and put in the filter, mounded with rich, dark coffee grounds. When I hear the burbling, the gasp of air, the hiss and sigh, and then smell that dark, biting euphony—it's only then that I know I'm going to be able to make it out the door on time. Before that, I'm in doubt.

Thank goodness for coffee.

I insist on clean, dark tastes, not a hint of bitterness. Full-bodied coffee with a resonance that lasts all morning. I don't like coffee to unnerve me. I don't want to slurp up acrid syrup at the bottom of the cup. No milk—just black. That's when you know a coffee, when you can drink it black. On top of that, I want my coffee to be organic and sold under fair-trade agreements. I drink enough of it that I want it to be right.

When I was younger, before I drank the stuff, the entire country suffered from a lack of coffee. When my parents made a pot of that dark liquid, it smelled thin, even to me. What did they use? Giant, five-pound cans of coffee, with metal sides and plastic lids, whatever rang up cheapest at the store at the time. When they opened the lid, I could smell the freezer burn on the ground coffee crystals, which were the color of caramel syrup. At the time, I thought that a cup of coffee looked like mud mixed with hot water, and I could not, for the life of me, figure out why people drank it. Luckily, I came into coffee-drinking consciousness when the rest of the country was waking up as well. I have never had to drink bad coffee.

On top of that, some instant coffees—the ones that come in little metal tins and promise the allure of a trip to Paris but really just taste like powdered milk with too much sugar and chemical additives—often contain gluten. For that reason alone, it's worth it to cultivate a taste for the finest coffee.

Okay, I know. Technically, coffee isn't a food. But it is sustenance, for those of us who drink it. And in order to make a great coffee ice cream, or a chocolate-espresso cake, I need the best-tasting coffee I can find. So do you.

Spend some money on dark-roasted, shade-grown, fair-trade coffee. You'll thank me in the morning, just after the alarm goes off.

10. local and independent

I know this is going to sound somewhat ludicrous, but believe me—
I am not alone in this. When I was growing up, I thought that companies *made* food. Oh, I know now that corporations process food,
package food, and, especially, sell food to a public with a raging
hunger-to-the-knees for substances that feel familiar in the mouth.
As an adult, I know what an enormous economic dynasty this is,
how much politics is involved, and how much we are directed in
what to eat because of multi-million-dollar marketing campaigns.

But when I was a kid, I honestly thought that those companies
owned that food. The Jolly Green Giant grew all the green beans.
Kraft created cheeses. General Mills *invented* cereal. Even though
we had an avocado tree in the backyard, and a pomegranate tree
dropped purple splotches on our cement patio, I did not fully realize
that food came from the earth or that someone had to harvest that
food for it to reach my hands.

When I was eight, my parents refrained from buying grapes from
the local supermarket for months on end. Sad to be without some
of the only fruit we ever had in the house, I asked my parents why
we couldn't just buy some green grapes. They informed me that
César Chávez had been advocating a boycott of table grapes for years
because the working conditions for the immigrant men and women
who picked them were horrifying. I became silent. I didn't know
that anyone even picked my grapes for me, much less thousands of
people, hunched over the fields all day long, sometimes doused in
pesticides, and suffering in poverty, their children unable to go to
school.

I have to admit that I lost my taste for grapes after that. Even
though I know that conditions for migrant workers are somewhat
better now, I rarely eat grapes. They feel tainted for me. Hearing
the story of how food truly came to my table made me wake up,
for the first time in my life. I had no idea that the food that arrived
in our grocery store came with more of a price than the tag on the
bottom.

Now, I'm not saying that all corporations are evil. But I will say this—when I have to call food companies to find out if I can actually eat the product I have in my hand at the grocery store, I run into problems with the biggest companies. First of all, I can never seem to reach a human being. Second, the ones I can reach equivocate, constantly, for fear of lawsuits or saying something the wrong way.

When I buy apples directly from the farmer at a Saturday morning market, I hear the story of his small farm east of the mountains, the effect the drought this summer had on his crop, how his nephew came up from Georgia to help him with the harvest and decided to try some organic techniques on his family's peach farm the next summer. That farmer is putting more in my hands than Cox Pippins and King Davids. He is giving me his life's work. I would much rather pay a bit more money to buy his food than buy in bulk from a multinational corporation.

Besides, his apples taste better than the ones in grocery stores.

There is a sign at my favorite farmers' market in Seattle: "Got bananas? We don't. Only Washington State produce is sold here." I love supporting small farmers and the people who truly care about the ethics and taste of foods.

But sometimes I have to go outside my area for great food. We don't make olive oil in Seattle. I don't want to live without olive oil. If I insist on only buying local, what do I do? What I learned, after I went gluten-free, is the joy of supporting small, independent businesses. My life has been made immeasurably better by a jar of chestnut honey from Tuscany, sweet and darkly enticing with the flavors of chestnut flowers half a world away. The man who makes this honey insists on doing everything by hand. He is also insistent on maintaining the environment in which the bees live. Everyone benefits by his being able to sell his honey to me (and you). Without this local company—and the Seattle-based importing company (Ritrovo) that brought it to me—I might have gone my entire life eating bland honey. And the reason I tried it in the first place is that my friend Seis put it into my hands in his store ten blocks from my door.

I consider that local also.

As you might imagine, that clear glass jar of sticky-sweet goodness cost me more than the honey-bear plastic jug would at the grocery store down the street. But I made that jar of honey last for nearly half a year. And I honestly remember every bite of it I ate.

Whether you are buying Sicilian olive oil, Drunken Goat cheese, champagne vinegar for salad dressings, or fresh dill to make pickles, where and how you buy your food matters. Find food producers you like, the ones who talk passionately about their products, their hands waving in the air. That food feels more enriching in your stomach than another jumbo box of cereal, made by an anonymous conglomerate. When you decide mindfully how to buy your ingredients, you will change your life.

Everything will taste better for it.

4

free to be you and me, gluten-free

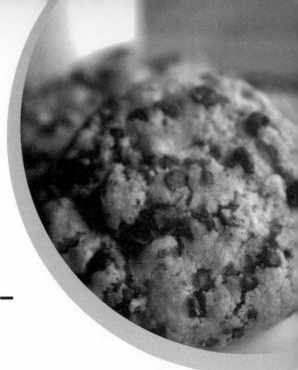

I have a confession to make: I used to suspect that people who claimed they had food allergies were making it up—or, at the very least, exaggerating.

How could anyone get so sick from a little wheat? Or some milk? A handful of walnuts? It seemed to me that people who ate wheat-free bread were just looking for attention. Granola heads. Pale people with no real vitality.

Watch out for what you doubt. It might just become you.

Part of my skepticism about food allergies was probably the influence of my parents. Take two kids with an agoraphobic mother, a father who teaches film and literature, put them in a home filled with books and fear under the surface, and what do you get? Two kids raised to believe they should be different than most people (translation: smarter and more educated) but not too different (translation: pretty much like their parents). Yoga, meditation, Ethiopian food, olive oil, Buddhist teachings—these were foreign concepts in my household.

But those practices and ideas are some of the foundations of the home I keep today. The older I grow, the less I feel I have to know. But I am sure of one thing now, after learning it the hard way: food allergies—as well as an autoimmune disorder triggered by gluten— are real.

I live in a country that prides itself on celebrating individuals. And yet we are deathly afraid of being different. It's as if our popular culture is dictated by a bunch of adults who have never left the seventh grade. When Kermit sang, "It's not easy being green," he was telling the truth. Step outside the preordained norm that no one ever speaks aloud—but that we all feel hovering around us—and you feel you ought to be ashamed.

According to recent estimates, 1 out of 100 people in the United States suffers from celiac disease. That's no small number. That makes at least 2 million people. It is not just those with celiac disease who need to avoid gluten. Hundreds of thousands of people have gluten sensitivity, gluten allergies, and wheat allergies. In addition, thousands of parents with autistic children are starting to put them on gluten-free and casein-free diets, which seem to alleviate some of the symptoms. The same is true for children with attention deficit disorder/attention deficit hyperactivity disorder and phenylketonuria, as well as adults with rheumatoid arthritis, schizophrenia, and diabetes. The medical field is just starting to understand how damaging gluten can be for millions of people.

According to the National Institutes of Health, only 3 percent of people with celiac disease have been diagnosed. As awareness of the disease grows, however, that number is increasing. Every week, I receive at least five e-mails from readers telling me that they were diagnosed with celiac disease since they started reading my Web site. My initial symptoms sounded so familiar that they recognized themselves. Every day, I receive dozens and dozens of e-mails from people who know that they must live gluten-free, but they are at a loss as to how to eat and live.

Eating gluten-free is not the latest fad in dieting. It is not a trendy choice. It is imperative.

Of course, there are millions more people who are trying to negotiate their lives without eating dairy, soy, or eggs. The parents of children with peanut allergies have to send their kids to birthday parties with epinephrine pens and a long list of what not to eat. Try living with a corn allergy—see if you can find a processed food that does not contain high-fructose corn syrup. (Did you know that Americans eat an average of sixty-three pounds of high-fructose corn syrup a year?) I have a dear friend who is so allergic to fish that he cannot be in the same room where fish has been prepared, or else his throat will swell up and he will have to be rushed to the hospital. He simply cannot go to restaurants. Imagine how isolated he feels.

We are not alone.

Think of it—most of us have some issue with food. And yet, somehow, we are seen as being on the fringes of society.

We can change this view. By living gluten-free successfully, and happily, for a couple years, there is one lesson I have learned clearly: the attitude I take toward this diet is just as important as the food.

No one who knows me now believes this—especially my students—but I used to suffer from mortifying shyness. As a bespectacled, chubby bookworm in Southern California in the 1970s and 1980s, I didn't talk much. I sat in the back of the classroom, fervently wishing that the teacher would not call on me. Forced to make speeches in English class, I flushed so red at the sound of my voice that I looked as though someone had slapped me repeatedly. It took all day for my nerves to soothe themselves. Sometimes, as I walked down the hallways of my school, I glanced up from my eyes-downward position to see groups of girls laughing with one another, their voices raised loudly enough that I could hear their conversations. I longed to be one of them: confident and free to speak.

When I was in the seventh grade, I decided that my big laugh was horrifying. Consciously, and with enormous effort, I forced myself to laugh a tiny "heh" when I found something funny. Literally, my laugh was no louder than those three letters look. How I thought that sound was less embarrassing than a real laugh, I don't know. But I made myself, out of a desperate desire to not stand out, laugh like that for six months. Need I say that those were the worst six months of my life?

Alongside my shyness stood my timidity at advocating for myself. For most of my childhood, I simply accepted what I was told to do, even if it didn't sit right in my gut. In my house, I was not allowed to insist on what I needed. My brain was trained to be submissive.

It took many years for me to become myself. We all have to leave the homes into which we are born and forge our own.

When I was seventeen, I decided to stop being shy. I had spent an entire year in London, with my family, without talking to anyone my own age. The loneliness finally proved a stronger force than the fear of talking to strangers. I pushed myself to talk to people three minutes longer than felt comfortable. By the time I hit my late twenties, I was a teacher, talking all day long. I had moved beyond the long arms of my mother, who would have kept me living in her house forever, if given her choice.

Four years in Manhattan did the trick even more. I will never forget my first day there. Standing in the middle of Times Square, I waited patiently at the corner for the light to turn green before I walked across the street. In Seattle, policemen gave tickets for jay-walking. I followed the rules. To my amazement, even though the light still stood fixed on red, dozens of people swarmed around me to enter the crosswalk en masse. Several of them glared at me for blocking their path. The light turned green, and I finally began walking, dazed as to what I should do. A yellow taxi tentatively entered the crosswalk, the driver trying to nudge the car past the pedestrians. Suddenly, a demure-looking woman with glasses—the archetypal librarian—threw her fist high into the air and slammed it down on the hood of the car. "The light's green, you fucker!" She walked on as though nothing had happened. I just stood and stared.

By the end of my time in New York, I had learned how to be

assertive. I never did slam the hoods of passing taxis, but I never again waited at a red light when the crosswalk was clear. People who have never lived there claim that New Yorkers are rude. Never. They are determined and assertive, and they know how to turn their shoulders to shimmy through a crowd fast. Because I lived in New York, I know how to ask for what I need, and without any fuss.

Life is too short. I have no time to waste.

This was all tremendous preparation for having to live gluten-free. In order to live well, I have to be assertive and clear. Even if people think I'm a picky eater or making something up, I have to stand up straight and ask for what I need. I have to move out of the corner and stand in the spotlight.

In order to keep myself safe, I constantly have to be on my toes. In grocery stores, I have to read every label before I buy anything. Even the brand I have been eating safely for months can suddenly change its ingredients, so I have to be meticulous enough to check, every time. In restaurants, I have to explain gluten and all the ways it can hide in foods and the dangers of cross-contamination to waiters and chefs. If the staff is not listening or is treating me with condescension, I have to have the guts to get up and leave. At family gatherings and holiday celebrations, I have to ask questions about the ingredients in the food that everyone made and pass up those plates with gluten, no matter how delicious they might look. As much as I appreciate the gesture of someone making homemade cookies, I have to turn them down, even if my hostess is offended.

start at home

You have just been diagnosed with celiac disease, and you are overwhelmed. What do you do?

Involve your friends and family. No one ever really lives alone. Three days after my diagnosis, my parents showed up at my home with new cutting boards, rolling pin, and toaster. Colleagues have left gluten-free cookie mixes on my desk. My friends, when they go to restaurants with me, are perfectly happy to order gluten-free meals, so we can sample and share our tastes. Luckily for me, the people in my life are happy to learn with me.

Avoid cross-contamination in the kitchen. You can prevent glutenization by being meticulous in the kitchen. Throw away your old wooden cutting board, because it can trap gluten in the surface, no matter how much you wash it. Do not use your regular toaster to toast the gluten-free bread, because the lingering bread crumbs will make you sick. Finally, keep the gluten-free food and the regular food in separate areas of the kitchen, and educate everyone about the dangers of double-dipping the spoon. Everyone will benefit from this information.

Make as much as you can from scratch. Celery, turkey, cranberries, and sweet potatoes in their pure form do not contain gluten. They never will. If you make everything from scratch, you will reduce any chance of accidentally ingesting gluten. Trader Joe's sells a boxed chicken broth that you might be tempted to buy for your gravy, but if you look at the ingredients list, it contains barley malt flavoring. One sip of that would set me back three days. Food we make from scratch will always taste better than food from a box. Take the time to do it right.

It's not as easy as substituting rice flour for wheat. If you throw together cinnamon rolls using your grandmother's recipe and simply substitute rice flour for enriched white flour, you are going to be sincerely disappointed. Gluten-free baking is an art and a science. It requires lots of experimentation and mistakes. Try to guide your life away from daily baked goods, if you can. Otherwise, there are a plethora of great gluten-free mixes that are available online and in health food stores. Even some large grocery chains are starting to carry gluten-free foods.

Be mindful. Walking through the grocery store on my first gluten-free shopping trip took me an hour and a half. When I checked out, I had only two bags of groceries to carry to the car. What took me so long? Scrutinizing all the labels. I need mustard. Is this one okay? For that first trip, I had a piece of paper with me on which I had written all the names for places that I had read where gluten can hide—such as hydrolized vegetable protein, maltodextrin, MSG, natural flavors, caramel color, distilled vinegar, and soy sauce. That didn't account for cross-contamination. Some of my purchases were easy—one-pound bags of various gluten-free flours; eggs; meats and seafood; fruits and vegetables. Essentially, if I shopped on all the outer edges of the store, with a little duck into the specialty baking section, I would be fine. However, on that shopping trip, I wanted something more. I wanted to find a bag of chips I could eat, some gluten-free pretzels, a couple of TV dinners that didn't have gluten. I was new at shopping gluten-free, and I wanted to ease in. However, I was struck by how aware I had to be, every time I picked up an item of food. Could this make me sick?

Never again can I simply pull something off a grocery store shelf and throw it into my basket without looking. That is a luxury of a bygone era.

Simply checking the labels is no longer enough, however. The knowledge of where gluten hides is constantly shifting. Luckily, it seems to be shifting in the favor of those of us who must avoid gluten, and anyone with food allergies. The Food Allergen Labeling and Consumer Protection Act of 2004 went into effect in January 2006. The act now requires food producers to name any of the top eight food allergens—wheat, dairy, peanuts, tree nuts, soy, corn, fish, and eggs—that might have been used in the making of their product. The label includes the official language: "manufactured in a facility that also manufactures wheat."

However, gluten is not on that list, because the government has not decided officially how to define gluten. There is a committee deliberating on that topic for the next two years. So, whenever I see wheat on a package, I know to put it down. However, if I don't see wheat, I still have to wonder.

I have also discovered that the places where people thought gluten hid—and thus were in all the official literature I consulted when first diagnosed—have undergone more scrutiny lately. As the awareness of celiac disease rises, so does our understanding. MSG manufactured in the United States no longer contains gluten. However, that means I need to be wary of any foods produced in Asia, of which I'm a big fan. Caramel color made in the United States no longer contains gluten, but I don't really drink anything with that in it anyway. It is now clear that distilled vinegar is gluten-free, which makes buying mustard and sauces much easier. (That is also why I can now drink Scotch.) Maltodextrin, I believe, is gluten-free if made in the United States, but I cannot seem to find an entirely clear answer on that one, so I just stay away.

In fact, the more I look at packaged foods, the less I want to eat them, even if they are gluten-free. Being mindful about what I read on the labels makes me run toward the fresh produce section.

However, even if I feel that I have figured out my brands, I still have to be mindful. One of my favorite brands of tortilla chips, made with organic corn and all the best intentions, was listed on the gluten-free list for Whole Foods. What could be better? When I was first diagnosed, I ate them with delight, excited to have something salty within easy reach. About eight months after going gluten-free, I started feeling slightly rotten. At first, I tried to console myself with the fact that it was winter, and thus everyone was burdened with a cold. But I listen to my body now, and I couldn't fool myself any longer. Something was wrong. I decided to look at my pantry with a beginner's mind, so I pulled down anything that could contain gluten. After an hour, only the tortilla chips were left. I had just started buying them again after months of not eating them. I logged onto the computer and searched through all the message boards for any mention of that brand. There it was—dozens of people confirming that they had suddenly grown sick on those chips. One reader reported that she had spoken with a representative of the company. He admitted that the company had changed some of the ingredients in the chips recently, as well as changing the methods by which the lines were cleaned. They were no longer calling their tortilla chips gluten-free. I immediately threw out the last bag I had in my house.

There is no question that living gluten-free requires enormous awareness and mindfulness. I have to ensure that every single bite of food I put in my mouth is free of gluten. No mindless nibbling, no "Oh, just this one." I have to be a detective, all the time.

There are two ways to approach this new way of being. I could whine and berate my fate, endlessly protesting that it just isn't fair. Or I could use it as an opportunity to be grateful. I'm serious—how much time of our lives do we waste in mindlessness anyway? Going gluten-free has forced me to become aware of the food I eat, the politics that bring it to my table, and the thousands of ways I can feed myself and be well.

Only use a packaged product if it says it's gluten-free. There are hundreds of products on the market that seem, from the list of ingredients, to not contain gluten. Even after you have figured out all the ways that gluten can hide, you can still make someone sick. I've done it to myself, because I wasn't careful. Some manufacturers are kind enough to say, "Manufactured in a facility that also manufactures gluten." When I read that, I put the food down. However, that's not all food producers. I have been glutenized by eating tortilla chips manufactured by a company that fries the chips in the same oil as gluten-filled products. Was it on the label? No. Why did I eat it? I just got stupid for a day. And I paid the price. Therefore, I would suggest that you only buy products that (a) say gluten-free on the box, or (b) you have confirmed yourself are gluten-free. This may seem draconian, but it is worth it.

Don't cheat. I am always struck by the numbers of people who write to me and admit, sheepishly, "You know, I cheat sometimes, and I always pay for it later." I have never been tempted to cheat. There is enough suffering in the world—I don't need to bring it on myself.

Ever since I was diagnosed with celiac disease, I have never once deliberately eaten something with gluten in it. In fact, for the first few months after my diagnosis, I had gluten nightmares, in which I dreamed I was eating bagels, or being chased by squadrons of crackers. Somehow, my brain processed the fact that gluten is poison to me. Would I "cheat" and drink some Drano? Because of my new life, those old gluten foods no longer appeal to me. I don't walk through a store and look longingly at everything I cannot eat.

Not everyone moves to this point of view immediately, however. A year ago, a reader left me a comment that I still remember. She had been diagnosed the year before and had lived strictly gluten-free for a few months. Then she faltered: "I had never felt so good, healthy, or energetic as I did when I was off gluten. I don't know how to go back to that. I feel like I am addicted to this crappy food I eat daily, this boxed stuff, and I hate it. I feel miserable, depressed, tired, arthritic (I'm 28), and constipated." Listen to that—she clearly feels terrible, and yet she keeps eating the prepackaged macaroni and cheese and the take-out pizza. This is a hard habit to kick, no question, especially when we have been raised since birth to believe that we should be eating processed foods and named labels.

The ability to commit to living gluten-free takes a psychological shift. It is a shift that must happen, however. How many people spend years mooning over the man who broke up with them, still wishing he was the one? Think of gluten as an abusive boyfriend. Sweep it away and open yourself to new experiences. If you are the type to cheat on your boyfriend, or cheat with some gluten when you have celiac, then find some help to deal with this behavior. This is no way to live.

Besides, if you cannot accept that you have to avoid gluten for the rest of your life, how do you expect everyone else in your life to understand it? It is hard to teach others how to cook for you when they see you stealing nibbles of the cookies laid out at the party. How will you clearly ask for a gluten-free meal at your favorite neighborhood restaurant if you hesitate when you talk about it and mumble so as not to make a fuss? I found that my life improved dramatically as soon as I was able to say, *I have celiac disease and I cannot eat gluten.*

Repeat that after me.

Don't you feel better already?

Why is any of this important?

Because for those of us who have celiac disease, an eighth of a teaspoon of gluten can make us sick for days. With a little care and mindfulness, we can all have a fabulous eating experience.

how to stand up for yourself

> I wish that I could be as strong and "shame-free" as you regard-
> ing food. I feel terrible when I get invitations to dinner or when
> I eat at a restaurant. I have to ask so many questions and people
> look at me like I must be a crazy hypochondriac or the pickiest
> eater ever. I am a pain to feed, so most of the time I'd rather
> cook for myself at home than feel like a burden to whoever is
> cooking. How do you get the point through to people that eat-
> ing things you're allergic to is bad, and allergies have nothing
> to do with being a picky eater???

This was a forlorn comment someone left on my Web site, after I wrote a post about dealing with Thanksgiving. Luckily, other read-ers bolstered this young woman, telling her to stand up for herself. She later wrote to me directly, thanking me. She had been changed by the conversation. However, hers is certainly not an isolated com-ment. In comments and other blogs and online discussion boards, gluten-free people profess that they are afraid of making a fuss.

It is clear that some of us who are diagnosed suffer from a crisis of conscience. In order to live well, we have to change our lives.

This is your life. Don't waste it. Being gluten-free may be difficult at times, but what life is without difficulties? I have never felt so good, or eaten so well, as I have since I went gluten-free. However, there are still times I am weary of it, times when I don't want to explain, once again, what will happen with my intestines if I eat that biscuit.

Once in a while, in spite of my best efforts, I am glutenized. This is my term for the times when I found out the hard way that an innocent-looking bite of food was cross-contaminated with gluten. I suffer for three days. However, those days of lethargy and pain give me enormous empathy for the person I used to be, the girl who always felt like this, the woman who suffered for years with no explanation. Every instance of cross-contamination that brings me down for days makes me remember how I have suffered and how many people are suffering that same way now. I come out of those instances even more resolved to stand up for myself.

Recognize the difference between being assertive and being aggressive. When I first found out that I had to be gluten-free and thought that eating in restaurants would be enormously difficult, I had only one image in my mind: Meg Ryan's character from *When Harry Met Sally.* That picky, persnickety woman drives everyone around her crazy when she orders food from a restaurant, everything on the side, heated to her liking, and dishes full of substitutions. Harry and the waiter roll their eyes when she is not watching. What an impossible woman.

That character—and hundreds of people like her—demand without being aware of what they are demanding. There's a feminine aggressiveness to it. *Cater to me,* that attitude seems to suggest. *Everything in the world must cater to me.* That's not what I mean by standing up for ourselves. Not at all.

When we are clear about what we need and ask for it simply, we save so much time. Let me tell you, as a teacher, just how frustrating it is to watch a student flailing in a discussion because she is afraid to be wrong when she expresses herself. "Umm, Ms. James, I don't know if this is right, I mean, someone might have said this already, and I could be wrong, but it seems to me, that, well, umm . . . was it red?" As she squirms in her seat and hesitates with every breath, every other student in the room is physically willing her to just spit it out. Some of them roll their eyes, the same way the waiter does in *When Harry Met Sally.* In the end, the poor dear ends up saying almost nothing. That shy student, afraid to make a fuss or say anything the wrong way, drew far more attention to herself than if she had just spoken up and briefly said her piece.

There is a big difference between being assertive and being aggressive. Aggressive is being pushy, with no compassion for what other people in the room are experiencing. It's not necessary to be aggressive to live gluten-free. Assertive, however, simply means being clear about what we need and then asking for it. If we are confident and strong in asking for what we need—in a restaurant, or in life— people will pay more attention and give us more respect.

Accept your sorrow. Sharon and I have been best friends since we were sixteen. Daily, we chatter and laugh through our cell phones, discussing every little detail of our lives. Most of the time, we are discussing what to eat. If Sharon and I have shared anything these past twenty-three years, it's food. We are both utterly devoted to food. We talk about meals in lavish detail and with multiple enthusiasms. We try recipes in separate states and report to each other about what worked. Sharon started me on fig balsamic vinegar, chai tea lattes, and chestnut honey on Pecorino Romano. We reminisce about meals: the sticky toffee pudding at Tea and Sympathy, sandwiches at Le Pain Quotidien, and pad thai at Thai Tom.

I always tease Sharon that when she is in the midst of an eyes-closed-it's-so-good breakfast at a little country bed-and-breakfast somewhere on a relaxed weekend away, she'll say, "Where are we going to have dinner?" Not lunch; not even dinner that night. She is wondering about dinner the next night—all the other meals in between are already planned and imagined.

When we reminisce about our epic cross-country road trip years ago, nearly every story we still tell each other has to do with food. The Italian beef sandwiches we ate in Chicago, hunched over the trunk of the rental car. (The splatterings stayed on that white car until a thunderstorm in Wyoming.) The milk shakes at the Yellowstone drugstore in Shoshone. The picnics and greasy breakfasts and cheese curds in Wisconsin. We are connected at the heart through our love for each other and our love of food.

When I was diagnosed with celiac disease and found out I could never eat gluten again, some essential part of my friendship with Sharon was lost. Now, when Sharon and I walk into tiny bakeries or little cafes, I breathe in the smell of the fresh-baked bread, and I feel a catch in my throat. Silly as it may sound, I feel genuine grief. Sometimes, it strikes me: my god, I'll never eat bread again.

I'm still not tempted to break bread with Sharon, however. I know exactly what gluten does to me, and it's no good. I see Sharon too infrequently anyway—she is in Los Angeles, trying to make a career as an actor, and I am in Seattle, teaching teenagers. During our precious visits, why would I want to spend my vacation feeling exhausted, cranky, wracked with headaches, and suffering from diarrhea for days? No thanks.

Instead of eating that treat as a way of being with her, I simply accept my sorrow. Instead of berating myself for feeling sadness, I allow it.

There's a quote from Albert Camus that I love, one that informs me every day: "The only way out is through." If you truly allow sadness to arise and don't push it away, it dissipates almost immediately.

One morning, during a visit to Los Angeles, Sharon and I were crossing the street on Sunset Boulevard. We had just ducked into a little bakery filled with delicate pastries and beautiful breads. Sharon wanted a little sweet after lunch. I knew I couldn't partake, but I was happy to go along. She bought two little lemon sugar cookies, crisp and slightly browned. There we were, walking slowly to the sidewalk. She bit into one of the cookies, and exulted, "Oh my god, this cookie is so good." She wasn't trying to make me feel bad. She just couldn't help it. Our entire lives of knowing each other, we've talked about our food. I could tell from her tone of voice just how good those cookies tasted.

For a moment, I felt lonely. But I recognized it, and I didn't try to stop the feeling. By the time we reached the curb, I was fine. There was so much goodness in the day. And besides, there I was at Sharon's side. What was I going to do—sulk the day away and waste the time with her? No, thanks. Instead, I felt it, and then I moved on.

After I flew home, I invented the following recipe for lemon olive oil cookies, because I was determined to have lemon cookies like those Sharon had. She spurred me to it. A vivid lemon olive oil from Sorrento, Italy, helped me create cookies that looked and smelled just like her cookies. Months later, when she was visiting me in Seattle, I made some for her. She swears they are better than those bakery cookies.

Lemon Olive Oil Cookies

1 cup sweet rice flour
1 cup tapioca flour
½ cup almond flour
1 teaspoon baking powder
½ teaspoon salt
¼ cup high-quality lemon olive oil
½ cup sugar
1 egg
¼ cup sour cream
3 tablespoons lemon juice
zest of 1 lemon
small bowl of sugar for rolling cookies

Combining. Mix the sweet rice flour, tapioca flour, almond flour, baking powder, and salt together. Set aside.

Creaming the liquids. Mix the olive oil and sugar together until well combined. Add the egg and blend. Slide in the sour cream and lemon juice. Mix until a cohesive mixture has formed.

Combining the dough. Slowly, fold the dry ingredients into the wet ingredients, a quarter cup at a time. (Incorporating the dry goods slowly helps with the texture of gluten-free baked goods.) Add the lemon zest at the last moment. The dough will be sticky. In fact, you might have dough all over your fingers by the time this process is done. Refrigerate the dough for at least 2 hours. (If you can stand to wait overnight, the dough will be even better.)

Preheating. Preheat the oven to 350 degrees F. Take the dough out of the refrigerator.

Rolling the dough. Form small balls with the sticky dough and roll each ball in a small bowl of sugar. Place the dough balls on a baking sheet covered with a Silpat or a layer of parchment paper.

Baking the cookies. Bake for approximately 10 minutes. The cookies will be soft at this point, but they will feel fully formed. These cookies are cakey in texture, so don't expect them to crisp up too much. Let them sit on the baking sheet for about 10 minutes.

Cooling the cookies. Carefully move the cookies to a cooling rack to rest for another 5 minutes, during which time they will harden.

Now, try not to eat them all in one sitting.

Makes 10 large cookies or 15 small ones.

Spread the awareness. Think of this: every time you stand up for yourself and say, "I need to eat gluten-free, and here's why," you are educating everyone you encounter about how to take care of the rest of us.

We aren't in this alone.

When I tell people that the name of my Web site is Gluten-Free Girl, or turn down a cookie and say why, or explain to a waiter how he can ensure I stay safe in his restaurant, every person has a similar response: "Oh, I know someone who has that." In all the time that I have been living gluten-free—and frankly, telling everyone I meet about the work I do—I have never run across a single person who says, "What? That's just weird." Instead, I feel more connected with people when I stand up for myself and tell them what is happening.

Every time I talk or write about this with ease, I am increasing awareness for everyone else. Perhaps some of you reading these words will realize that you might have celiac disease and decide to get tested.

Every one of us can play a part, simply by telling our story.

how to travel gluten-free

Since I have found out I cannot eat gluten, I have traveled to Los Angeles (twice), New York, Alaska (twice), and Tucson, Arizona. Each time, I have laughed with friends, gained a hundred stories, and experienced the world in a different way for being out of my home. Each time, I have successfully stayed healthy and gluten-free.

When I'm at home, I no longer worry about eating gluten-free. After all, nothing with gluten comes into my house. When I step through the door of my upstairs apartment, I breathe easy. Here, I just feel alive. Here, I'm just thinking about what's in season. Should I make millet or quinoa? Seafood or chicken? Soup, spontaneously? Ah, these are the decisions I love.

But traveling gluten-free can be a bit of a trial. After all, every coffee shop serves muffins, scones, and cookies. Certain restaurants beckon with bread or pizza. Airports are simply a nightmare.

However, traveling gluten-free can be done, and with enormous flair. If you have to eat gluten-free and you're planning a trip, here are a few lessons I have learned. I hope they make your life easier.

Plan ahead. Before I went gluten-free, whenever I went traveling, I always packed my suitcases the morning of my trip. Even when I was going to London for six months on a 6 A.M. flight, I was packing at midnight. But those days are over now.

If I forget to pack my own toothpaste, I just can't be sure that the friend I'll be staying with will have gluten-free toothpaste. If I forget my prescription ibuprofen for my broken foot—the one that took forty-five minutes for the pharmacist to find out from the manufacturer that the pills are gluten-free—then I have to rummage through my friend's medicine cabinet. If I find that I can't take the brand that's there, I have to be in pain.

Long before the day I leave, I also go online to some of the celiac forums and message boards and put up a question about traveling. Hey, I'm coming to your town. Where do you eat? What restaurants would you trust? Are there farmers' markets anywhere nearby? Anyplace I should definitely avoid? People are enormously helpful on these forums. I've had dozens and dozens of questions answered there.

Pack your lunch. I can guarantee you this: if you are going through an airport, there will be nothing for you to eat. Airports are filled with bad food: greasy, breaded, and overpriced. But you'll find, fairly quickly, that everything in airport stores and restaurants seems to have gluten in it. There are a few possible exceptions. Smoothie shacks seem to be sprouting up these days, and they probably don't have gluten. But you never know. And unfortunately, the awareness level about gluten at airport concession stands isn't high. It probably isn't worth the risk to eat anything at the airport.

What about the food on the airplane? Well, since the airlines seem to have cut down on their meal service in general, it's nothing but the little bags of pretzels and the roasted peanuts. Pretzels? Obviously not, but even the peanuts are suspect. Some roasting methods for nuts involve gluten. However, you're not missing much. When was the last time you actually enjoyed food at the airport or while sitting hunched into a narrow airline seat? Instead, pack yourself a beautiful lunch for the trip. While everyone else is looking miserable and wishing those packages of peanuts had been larger, you can pull out pieces of sashimi, some gluten-free cornbread, or a smoked salmon salad with quinoa. Or at the least, enjoy a gluten-free energy bar and some kiwi fruit.

Look for gluten-free bakeries and restaurants. I have discovered after going gluten-free that most of the people who make gluten-free foods make great food. They all started with a sense of urgency, a real desire to make food that lingers in the memory with unexpected pleasure. Those foods come with fervency. A woman starts baking gluten-free cookies in her home. Everyone remarks, "These are fantastic. I wouldn't even know they are gluten-free!" Driven forward by the sense of joy her food is giving people, she starts delivering to local coffee shops. And then she decides to open her own bakery.

With the rise in awareness of celiac disease, and the numbers of people who must eat gluten-free, many big cities in the United States have a gluten-free bakery or restaurant. When you are in the unfamiliar territory of a city you don't know, it is an enormous comfort to walk into a restaurant where you know you will not grow sick.

Bring a cell phone. I can't believe that I'm advocating cell phones. It took me years to buy one, and then only reluctantly. I dislike the way people talk about the most personal details of their lives on a city bus or shout in the middle of a store. We are becoming boorishly behaved because of this new technology.

However, if you can't eat gluten and you are traveling, they are remarkably handy. How? Well, say you'd like to eat some scrumptious packaged dessert with your friend. You look at the list of ingredients, and it looks fine. But how do you know? Well, every company seems to have an 800 number on the back of the package. Whip out your cell phone and call customer service. Tell the representative that you are on the verge of purchasing the company's fine product, but you need to know that you can eat it first. You'd be amazed at the alacrity with which companies will search for that information for you. If the company is reluctant to tell you or is ignorant of the information you request, that's good for you to know as well.

Give yourself a treat. All that being said, you deserve a little treat when you're traveling. I seek out gourmet stores and farmers' market. When the money allows, I buy myself tidbits of food I wouldn't normally eat. A Vietnamese coffee in the middle of the day. Sea salt caramels. Persimmons. A Drunken Goat cheese from Spain. At the Casbah Café in Los Angeles, I bought a package of dried apricot paste from Syria, a few moments after Sharon bought the lemon cookies I could not eat. I had never eaten it before, but now I am addicted. The morning I returned, I tried a small square of it with a semisoft goat cheese rolled in basil. That singular taste was far more memorable than one of those cookies would have been.

how to eat in restaurants gluten-free

In the nearly four decades before I found out I had to stop eating gluten, I loved eating in restaurants. From fresh-made manicotti in New York to sushi in Seattle, I ate in restaurants as an entertainment, an adventure, and a chance to learn everything I could about food. Without eating in restaurants, my palate might have remained as narrow as it had been when I was a kid.

When I was diagnosed with celiac disease, and I read the advice of countless experienced gluten-free people, I resigned myself to what seemed like an inevitable fact: I would never eat in a restaurant again. Between my memories of pizza and pasta and the warnings of people screaming about the dangers of cross-contamination, I just could not see how I could eat in a restaurant without growing sick. In my mind, I foresaw a healthy life a bit bereft of innovation. *There goes Paris*, I thought. *I'll never have another meal in Italy.* And how could I ever return to my favorite restaurants in New York City? However, it all seemed worth it. I would have done anything to have my health clear and my energy moving. So, I gave up restaurants.

Thank goodness I got over that.

For the first three months after I went gluten-free, I did not set foot in a restaurant. It took my intestines that long to recover so that I could eat meat and dairy again. Whenever I could add in new foods, I felt as if the world had opened up again. I did not need chefs cooking for me. Just being able to eat was enough.

However, after my health improved and I had done enough research and living to feel that I had the hang of being gluten-free, I knew that I could not stay in a place of fear anymore. I missed Vietnamese pho, injera bread, sashimi so fresh I could see through the thinly sliced fish, and the scintillating flavor combinations that a creative chef can invent to make a dish that I never could have imagined. Eating only beans and rice or sautéed salmon just wasn't enough for me.

In the past two years, I have eaten beautiful, exquisite foods that

I could never have made by myself, in some of the best restaurants in Los Angeles, New York, Alaska, and Seattle. I cannot imagine the pallid nature my life would have taken on if I had not eaten these foods.

Los Angeles. A sweet corn salad, with black, wrinkled olives; fresh tomatoes; and tuna. A warm duck breast with balsamic vinegar and a side of perfectly sautéed spinach. Seared ahi tuna drizzled with parsley pesto, with a side of roasted eggplant and wild mushrooms.

New York. Chicken sausages and caramelized apples in Cobble Hill. Marinated mozzarella balls from Murray's Cheese Shop on Bleeker Street. The softest, falling-off-the-bone lamb tagine I have ever eaten on St. Mark's Place. Lentil stew and a great bottle of wine in Nolita. Even a couple of hot dogs from Gray's Papaya, without the bun, on my last day in the city, when I was already feeling sad about having to return home.

Alaska. Massive Dungeness crab legs, dunked in warm garlic butter. Spicy tuna rolls at a tiny sushi place forty feet from the port in Sitka, the freshest fish I have ever eaten. Prawns, hand-caught by the chef, thrown on the grill and tossed on my plate.

Seattle. Thin, crackling slices of pork jowl, crunching among tiny brown lentils, along with small shreds of grilled radicchio and arugula. A towering plate of julienned apple pieces, pomegranate seeds, slices of salty prosciutto, and dots of bright green pesto. Pan-roasted sweetbreads, sautéed at such high heat in a cast-iron skillet that they had a little crust, with a veal stock reduction sauce. Braised baby short ribs, with crispy polenta, fried avocadoes, and a poblano–sour cream sauce.

You see? There is no deprivation in living gluten-free.

However, there is no avoiding the fact that every time you eat in a restaurant, you are taking your chances. But if you choose your restaurants well, ask lots of questions, and gently pester every employee in the place (because it's your right, and you should), then you should be in pretty good shape. Here are some of the ways that I have eaten gluten-free in so many restaurants, in cities across the country.

Go to restaurants where they truly care about the food. Many gluten-free people either refuse to eat out or go only to enormous chain restaurants that have a few entrées marked as gluten-free. More power to those chains for trying, but I never would have eaten at a chain restaurant before this diagnosis, and I'm not going to now. I much prefer small, intimate places with gourmet sensibilities. With a small restaurant, renowned for its fresh, seasonal tastes, you are also going to find chefs and waiters who know food and care about what they do. I love restaurants where the waiters feel like partners in the process, rather than people run off their feet. I also adore restaurants that are warm in decor, well-lit, and have about fifteen tables. Those are restaurants that would never cook with anything prepackaged. They know what gluten is. They will direct you correctly. You may pay a little more at restaurants like this, but the food will be far better than at a slightly cheaper chain. Don't you want your eating experience to be memorable?

Choose cuisines that tend to be naturally gluten-free. Don't go to a pizza place and ask for anything gluten-free. Don't go to a cheap pasta place and sulk because you can only eat a salad. Branch out. Try foods you wouldn't normally eat, in cuisines that don't use much gluten in the first place.

Indian cuisine employs alternative flours, like chickpea, on a regular basis, and they have for hundreds of years. Avoid the naan and stick to the papadum (traditionally made with chickpea or lentil flour). Ask if they use anything like asafoetida that could contain gluten, and then dig in.

Thai food, with its use of rice and rice noodles, is one of the most illuminating foods in the world, layered with tastes and vibrant in the mouth. Just ask about their use of soy sauce, fish sauce, and oyster sauce. Bottled sauces can contain wheat. If you find a truly authentic restaurant, however, they probably make their own sauces. Some Thai restaurants use a flavoring agent called Maggi sauce, which contains gluten. Find a Thai restaurant where the waitstaff speak English well enough to take care of you. Ask that they use a freshly cleaned wok to cook your meal, and then you can eat.

Mexican food, especially the restaurants that make food that Mexicans like to eat, serve corn tortillas. Wheat flour doesn't appear often. You still have to ask. You can't assume. But you're far more likely to find something you can eat on the menu if you go Mexican.

Good seafood restaurants are likely to have something for us, pretty easily.

Vegetarian and vegan restaurants are more aware of food allergies than traditional restaurants. In my experience, waiters and chefs in vegetarian restaurants are likely to be aware of what gluten is and where it lurks. They're pretty universally friendly.

Then there is Vietnamese food, which is one of my favorites. On a cold winter day, there is nothing I crave more than a big bowl of pho—rice noodles floating in a beautiful broth, slender slivers of beef, crunchy sprouts, basil leaves, and peppers so hot they make my friend Pete sweat out of his forehead. (Those are optional.)

There are so many options.

Plan ahead. If I know that I want to eat at one of the best restaurants in Seattle, I call ahead. I let them know about my gluten issue, and I walk them through what I cannot eat. Usually, I make the reservation for a time I know will be less busy than 7:30, the time when chefs are up to their ears in orders. I like eating at 5:30, or at 9—the waiters can give me more attention than they can when things at the restaurant are hectic.

Be solicitous and meticulous about your condition. I am going to have far more success at eating gluten-free if I am friendly and open and ask for my waitperson's help rather than being demanding or anxious. It sets the tone of reciprocity right away. The spiel always begins with a smile and is followed by, "I'm really sorry to be a bother, but . . . ."

Tell the waitstaff what you need to avoid to stay healthy. Ask for it in a clear, specific tone. This communicates to the waitstaff, right away, that you know what you are doing and that you are trying to help them. This is the last part of the spiel I always say at a restaurant:

". . . and if I get even a speck of gluten, I will get really sick in your restaurant." It is that last phrase—*in your restaurant*—that will capture the attention of your waitstaff, and thus the chef.

Thank your waitperson and chef if they are kind, and tip well. A few kind words about the service makes the people who serve you feel good about their work. I have been given free oysters, glasses of wine, and gluten-free desserts, on the house, for being such a thoughtful customer who appreciated my waiter or waitress.

I have always been a generous tipper, because many of my close friends have been waitresses and chefs. However, after I started eating gluten-free at restaurants, I have been extra generous. Why? I want the people at that restaurant to associate gluten-free customers with generosity. I want to pave the way for the next table full of people who are eating their first gluten-free restaurant meal in six months.

Go back. If you had a successful experience eating gluten-free in a restaurant, return, again and again. As exciting and necessary as it is to try new places, there is nothing like the comfort of having a familiar place, where the waitstaff and chef know your face. After all, every time I eat in a restaurant and leave with a contented stomach, I am a happy, gluten-free girl.

how to survive the holidays gluten-free

I had every intention of having a gluten-free Thanksgiving the November after my celiac diagnosis. Every Thanksgiving of my life before that one was spent with my stomach overly full, my throat constricted, my head pounding from the pain, and a general feeling of malaise. We all overeat on Thanksgiving, right? I assumed that is why I always felt like such a dragged-out, run-over specimen of a being for most of Thanksgiving day.

Now I know that the discomfort of years past was gluten. After my diagnosis, for the first time, I would have an entirely gluten-free Thanksgiving.

I tried.

My brother and sister-in-law had bought a fresh turkey, and they decided to roast it in a plastic poultry bag. As I was making my gravy with cornstarch, I watched my dear brother take the turkey out of the oven. I remarked on how lovely and brown it looked. And then I stared at the bag.

"Hey, Andy, what's that white stuff in the bag?" I asked him.

"Oh, it's flour. The manufacturers suggest you throw a couple of tablespoons of flour in there to make sure the skin doesn't stick," he said, with no hint of recognition in his voice.

I stared at him.

And then he looked at me, his eyes growing wide, and said, "Oh, shit."

He and my sister-in-law had put flour on the turkey. The one part of the Thanksgiving dinner most likely to be gluten-free was now floured up.

My brother and sister-in-law know all about the gluten-free thing, since they both read my Web site. I know they never had any intention of shutting me out of the Thanksgiving turkey. But that's how hard this is. Even the people who care about us sometimes just don't make the connection. And then we gluten-free folks have to go without. Again.

In the flurry of finishing my gravy and laying out the cranberry chutney, I didn't notice that Andy had set my pan of pale gluten-free stuffing and his pan of toasted-brown regular stuffing side by side. Or that they were in the exact same glass pans. But I did notice, when I went into the kitchen to grab seconds, that someone had put the spoon from the regular stuffing in mine, by mistake. I looked at it, in horror. Had that happened before I took my first serving? I tried to take a spoonful from the other side, with a new spoon, but it probably wasn't enough of a precaution.

An hour after dinner, I started feeling exhausted. Bloated. That horrible sinking feeling of eating too much. I had to lie down on the couch. My face felt hot. I could feel the headache rising. And my gut began reacting, almost immediately. Somehow, I had ingested some gluten.

Why didn't I make a fuss and make all my own dishes, color-coded, in spite of my brother's wish to treat the entire family to food? I was learning. There are so many gluten-free lessons to learn. This is a path, a practice, and a continually unfolding journey.

However, I was sick all that weekend. Terrible flashes of headaches. Enormous strains of lethargy. Foggy brain. Significant grumblings in the intestines, and more. The old pain in my side. A fullness in my stomach, rising up through my throat, almost choking me. Bloatedness in every part of me. Joint pain. And no appetite. All because of a cross-contaminated spoon.

That weekend cured me. I vowed I would never spend another holiday sick again. From then on, I followed my own way home.

The winter holidays in this country have become an inexorable march toward consumption and gaudiness. How many presents can you buy in one fell swoop? Quick—put the lights up on the house! We must make dozens of cookies, right now. Never mind that this consumerism has nothing to do with the spirit of any of the holidays around the darkest time of the year. This is what we do. We celebrate the holidays, damn it.

That compulsion to make everything the same as the year before, and the need to have it be as perfect as a Martha Stewart magazine layout, sweeps up most of us, in one way or another. But for those of us who have celiac disease—and must eat gluten-free in this gluten-saturated time of the year—that time of the year can be a minefield. (I am certain this must be true for anyone with food allergies, as well as vegetarians and vegans, so this is quite a large number of us.) I don't miss gluten. But I do miss the sugar cutout cookies I made every year for over a decade. I miss gingerbread men and my mother's cinnamon rolls on Christmas morning. I'll never have them again. It's okay to feel a little bit of mourning.

Every year, the e-mails I receive from readers triple in November and December. They are all heartfelt and pleading. One young woman told me that she had volunteered to make Christmas dinner for everyone in her family. Could I create gluten-free versions of all the treats the family wanted to eat? I've had requests for cinnamon rolls, mincemeat pie, stuffing, and gluten-free gravy. Everyone, it seems, wants to eat exactly what he or she ate as a child—before the celiac diagnosis—and have it taste exactly the same.

It will never taste the same. No matter how good your pumpkin pie recipe with a gluten-free crust, it will never taste like the pie you ate as a child. It could taste even better. But it won't taste the same.

In my opinion, Thanksgiving could use some shaking up. Here was my biggest surprise during my first gluten-free Thanksgiving: even if I hadn't been glutenized, I would not have enjoyed the meal much. The traditional Thanksgiving meal is a plate of food that all tastes pretty much the same: starchy, mashed, salty, and full of flour. Any vegetables served are clotted with sauces. What other meal would feature mashed potatoes and sweet potatoes? After six months of cooking with fresh foods and an open mind, I just wasn't that interested in the traditional dinner. In the end, the food I enjoyed most was the butternut squash I had roasted with sea salt and olive oil in the early afternoon, just enough to tide us over until the big dinner. That is the taste that stuck with me.

So, let the holidays be a time of opening and discovery, instead of shutting down.

Mix up the traditions. Years ago, when I was a teenager, my father told us about a class he had taught the day before Thanksgiving. He asked his students their families' food traditions, which led to a spirited discussion of the merits of different kinds of stuffings. One of his students had a different story, however. She said that her parents were Italian immigrants, and they made an enormous Italian feast for Thanksgiving: pastas, roasted meats, antipasti platters, fresh mozzarella. My father said that her description made him hungry. Would we want to try that? As one, my brother and I shouted, "No!" We wanted our traditions, and that was that.

But you know what? I'd be more than willing to try it now, as long as the pasta was gluten-free. Isn't this holiday a chance to celebrate life with family and friends with food? Who says that it has to be a glossy roasted turkey with bread stuffing spilling out of its cavity? Why not curried carrot soup? Black cod? Roasted duck? Seared tofu? Why not make it a menu of all the foods you have come to love since you went gluten-free? Instead of calling it Thanksgiving, or insisting on the same meal you had every Christmas Eve, why not call it a celebratory feast? Offer up rich, decadent foods with enormous bodies of flavor. Swiss chard gratin. Cassoulets. Braised lamb. Brussel sprouts in browned butter. Sweet potato puree. Crisp salads with goat cheese and pomegranate seeds. Have a table full of twenty dishes, and then ask everyone to dig in. Would anyone feel a lack of gratitude at that?

Offer to cook dinner yourself. I know this might seem like a lot of work, but it will make everyone in the family happy, and you will be assured of eating gluten-free food. Sure, it means a day of cooking, but there is almost nothing better than the simple joy of feeding people we love. If you cannot cook the entire dinner, then at least offer to make the parts of the meal that usually involve gluten. Make pies and rolls and a loaf of gluten-free bread for stuffing.

Teach your family about cross-contamination. Sit down with everyone, long before the big day, and explain all the ways that gluten can hide. The holidays are supposed to be infused with gratitude. Your family can express their gratitude by cooking gluten-free food. You will feel enormous gratitude if you can eat an entire meal that won't make you sick.

Find a way out, if your family won't help. Let's hope that your family will choose you over their traditional stuffing. However, if you encounter truculence and passive-aggressive behavior, have your own holiday. Gather all your best and most supportive friends—the family you chose—and cook a huge meal together. If your family feels miffed, tell them that you would like to join them next year, if they can support you. Or, if you want to still join in with your family, have an early dinner with your friends and join your family for coffee and wine at the end of the night. I imagine, however, that your clear explanation of the situation—as well as the possibility of your not arriving for the holiday—will help your family to help you.

Just say no to gluten. 'Tis the season when people are tempted to cheat. That spoonful of stuffing isn't worth three days of feeling sick. Those cinnamon rolls will never be worth the price you'll pay in your gut. Make a new tradition of staying well throughout the holidays. You owe it to yourself.

If you are mourning the loss of traditional dishes, please remember this: there is more at stake here than your grandmother's stuffing. As a lovely woman named Wendy wrote to me one Thanksgiving, "My daughter was diagnosed in April of this year. This is our first holiday season with a healthy girl!" Isn't the celebration of that far more important than eating the exact same foods you have eaten all your life?

Let this holiday be a true day of gratitude. Let's eat well and celebrate.

5

vegetarians, please avert your eyes

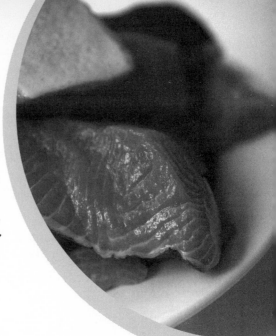

At one point in my life, I thought I would never eat meat again.

The thin red juices at the bottom of the polystyrene package? They made me feel a little queasy. After I had taken an anatomy and physiology class in high school, cutting into chicken breasts always reminded me of dissecting frogs. Even though I worshipped the LA Dodgers when I was eleven and twelve—and showed my devotion by sitting in front of the television every day, listening to Vin Scully call the game, while I ate a Dodger dog—I always felt dubious about the nature of hot dogs.

Feeling squeamish about meat made it a little difficult to eat in my house. Oh sure, I could have sugary cereals for breakfast, but on weekends we had packaged sausage links with our pancakes. If we had spaghetti sauce from a jar or goulash with a seasoning packet, we needed ground beef. Because my mother had grown nauseated while cooking it when she was pregnant with my brother, she made me sauté the ground beef until it was uniformly beige-brown. All meat was well done to the point of desiccation in our house. Taste didn't really matter as much as not dying. When I needed a chair to see into the skillet to stir with the plastic spatula, I felt special because I had been assigned this task. By the time I was a teenager, I started to feel a little sick of it.

For dinners almost every summer night, my father barbecued meat for us, fulfilling his male cooking duties. Hamburgers came in frozen stacks, wrapped in plastic, with a texture like insulation for walls. Those patties had a waffle pattern already stamped into them, and they tasted vaguely like the half-beef/half-soy burgers they served at the school cafeteria. By the time my father lifted them off the grill, they were gray. We smothered the burgers in ketchup and smashed the white-flour buns down upon them. Barbecued chicken came slathered with bottled sauce, neon orange flecked with red, overly sweet and smoky. I won't lie—I attacked the drumsticks like Henry VIII. My mother made homemade potato salad, and my fingers dripped splatters of barbecue sauce onto the eggy-yellow goodness. However, after years of eating that dinner, I started to crave a new sensory experience. That bottled-sauce chicken always tasted exactly the same as the last time I had eaten it. On special occasions, my father grilled up T-bone steaks the size of Nebraska on a map of the Midwest. They lay recumbent on our plates, dwarfing the cobs of corn and pats of butter. Because they were charcoaled almost past recognition, I sought out the little pockets of fat on the back that crackled with taste. Increasingly, those few bites would have been enough for me, but there was nothing much else to eat.

Meat was the sole, dominating influence of our dinners. Everything else was garnish, like the sprigs of warm parsley that arrived on plates in restaurants when we ate out. Everything other than the meat seemed insignificant, an afterthought. Meat was not a flavoring; it was a way of life.

It probably didn't help that food safety was my mother's number-one priority—everything else was secondary. Her panics about any perceived threat took a thousand different forms in our lives. But in food, it meant one thing: overdone meat. Turkeys arrived at the Thanksgiving table so dry that the skin around the drumstick crackled like old parchment paper. Every year, she made us put our noses into the raw turkey and take deep whiffs before she put it in the oven, urging us to ferret out any suspect poultry smells. One year, she threw out the turkey because she insisted that it smelled like aspirin. We ate only stuffing and mashed potatoes for dinner.

We rarely ate in a "fine dining" restaurant, despite my father's persistence in remembering the one fabulous Italian meal he ate before I was born. We didn't have that much money because Dad was a teacher and Mom stayed at home with us. So, when we did eat out, we went to kid-friendly fast-food restaurants. I must have eaten nearly a ton of Quarter-Pounders at McDonald's, acres of enchiladas at Del Taco, and a fair amount of shredded beef sandwiches at Arby's. Summer afternoons at the ocean ended with the meatball entrée at the Spaghetti Factory in Newport Beach. Lunches at Disneyland meant beef tacos with shredded cheese at Casa del Fritos, a plastic re-creation of a Mexican taco stand. The only time I didn't eat meat in a restaurant was when I ordered the enormous platter of overly creamy fettucine alfredo at Marie Callender's. That—and the Frogger game my brother and I played in the smoking lounge as we waited for a table—is my main memory of restaurant dining when I was a child.

Nearly every day for lunch, before I was sixteen, I ate a sandwich with squishy white bread and a slice of meat from the plastic variety meat pack. The only variation was the form of meat I ingested each lunch. Would it be the Cotto salami, pale pink with little pockets of white fat? When I was home for lunch, on the weekends or during the summer, I sometimes made fried bologna sandwiches. I'd plug in the electric griddle and throw a couple of slices of bologna on its black surface. When the bologna slices buckled and bubbled, I turned them over onto the other side. I had white bread with margarine waiting, along with a slice of American cheese. Sliding the fried bologna onto the white slice, I threw it all back onto the grill and let the margarine darken in little brown pockets on the white bread. Voilà! A grilled-cheese sandwich with fried bologna. I ate all the meats in that flat pack that my mother threw into her grocery cart every week, except the liverwurst. Unlike Leopold Bloom, I did not relish eating the internal organs of beasts and fowls. That thought was just plain disgusting.

More and more, however, even the most basic meats started to seem disgusting. At sixteen, I found *Laurel's Kitchen*, and I became determined to become a better person and live my life without meat. It was, of course, a colossal disaster. My entire diet seemed to consist of soggy veggie burgers, required cottage cheese, lots of mushy apples, and carrots. This, along with the glare of my mother, who thought me weird, persuaded me to give up my attempt to become a vegetarian.

I went back to vegetarianism, however, when I was in college. As is true for many college students, I went through a fervent feminist phase, an ardent environmentalist stage, and a virtuous vegetarian diet. All of them stuck, in one form or another, for years afterward. In classes on social thought and ethics, I pondered the need to eat meat when so many people in the world were starving. Like many young Americans, I read John Robbins's *Diet for a New America* and Upton Sinclair's *The Jungle*. My love of animals, my desire to save the world, and—frankly—the guilt instilled in me at an early age made me turn vegetarian.

Of course, at the college cafeteria, a vegetarian meal meant overcooked broccoli and ranch dressing from the salad bar, commercial veggie burgers on white-flour buns, and peanut butter and jelly sandwiches. I still didn't feel good.

Luckily, by the time I moved to Vashon Island in my twenties, I had made friends who knew how to cook. I shopped at the Saturday farmers' market, and I asked everyone I knew to give me vegetarian cookbooks for presents. Slowly, my taste buds expanded. Avid, as always, I worked hard to combine my proteins and to eat well. It was becoming a vegetarian that made me a real cook. No longer able to rely solely on meat and potatoes, I was forced to find new flavors and spices before hidden from me. Soy sauce splashed in my stir-fries. Fresh dill settled in among the new potatoes steaming on my stove. I ate baklava with wild honey, pesto with fresh basil grown in my friend Tita's garden, and Thai peanut sauce on spicy noodles.

Everything started to taste more alive than when I had eaten only packaged and processed meats.

Of course, I was still eating a mostly gluten diet, but I didn't know the damage it was doing to me then.

However, I still secretly longed for meat sometimes. Oh, I felt sure that I was doing the right thing, intellectually. How could I be a better person than by being a vegetarian? I was saving the animals, saving the earth, saving myself from cooking ground beef. In my mind, it was clear: I *should* be a vegetarian. And yet . . .

When I went over to Tita's house for dinner and she was barbecuing chicken with her homemade sauce—twenty different ingredients, all of them fresh—my eyes always traveled toward the grill as we ate our salads. The smell of Julie's pasta dishes with tiny slices of beef tenderloin was more appealing than my pasta with cheese. And sometimes, to my surprise, I even missed hot dogs.

The fact is that not all the meat of my childhood had been bad. My mother's chicken enchiladas may have been made with canned chiles, but damn, they were good. Her chili may have been topped with crushed Fritos, but I was still delighted when she served it for dinner. And in my hometown, Greene's Delicatessen served pastrami sandwiches that would have put the Carnegie Deli to shame. I can still taste the Reuben sandwiches my mother made for my brother's birthday dinner, with crusty rye bread, sauerkraut, thick slices of Swiss cheese, and pastrami from Greene's. My mouth is watering now, just thinking of it. The good food and meats of my childhood kept nudging into my memory.

I kept on with my vegetarian mission, but inside, in secret, was a woman wanting to eat meat.

Throughout it all, I continued to eat fish. The only fish we ate in my house came breaded, in stick form, and from the freezer. My mother shocked us the first time we went to McDonald's and she ordered one of their new creations, the Filet O'Fish. (Why was a breaded fish sandwich slathered in tartar sauce supposed to be Irish?) Of course, she demanded it dry, and cooked well, and everything on the side. But still—fish instead of meat? I ate fish and chips in London, the year I lived there as a teenager, every other day. Those tastes of fish—breaded and fried though they may have been—taught me that protein didn't always have to taste like blood and charcoal.

And so, when I was a vegetarian, I was really a pescetarian. When I was living on an island off Seattle in my midtwenties, it felt like a travesty to not eat the wild salmon that showed up in the market. My friend Julie made grilled halibut for me on one of our summer deck days, and I was hooked. Clams and mussels showed up in the soups of humble restaurants on the island, and I slurped them all up. The variety of tastes floored me—the rich oiliness of salmon tasted nothing like the flat blandness of sole. Deprived of good fish for my entire life, I started eating every fish dish in my sight. My body liked it—I was finally eating enough protein. (Sometimes I forgot to combine my beans and rice, because I really didn't know how to cook beans with any flavor yet.) Eating fish always seemed to make me feel more clearheaded and filled with energy. Now, I realize, it is because I didn't bread and fry the fish in flour. In those meals, I ate fish, rice, and vegetables. For a brief, shining time, I had a life without gluten.

Something started to plague me. If I was eating fish, why was I not eating meat? Why was a salmon less worthy to me, in my mission to save the animals, than a cow? I felt like a hypocrite, especially because I was still nursing those secret longings to nibble on a pastrami sandwich sometimes. Not knowing what to do with this conundrum, I just shoved it in the back of my mind.

When I moved to Manhattan, I tried to be a vegetarian. However, I found it more difficult to be a pescetarian than I had when I lived on that island on the West Coast. In New York, I was living on the Upper West Side, going to graduate school in the Village, tutoring students on the Upper East Side, and writing in every spare moment that I could find. I tried to combine my rice and beans, make soup from scratch, and dwell in the tranquil land of healthy eating, but it felt impossible in that pulsing, frantic city. Within a few weeks,

I relented and ate the way every other New Yorker I met seemed to eat—on the run, a sandwich from the bodega in hand, lunch out with friends, a pint of Ben and Jerry's in bed at night. Because of all the running down subway steps, shuttling between neighborhoods, and living one eye-opening day after another, my body must not have been receiving the proper nutrition. My mother was finally right—I needed more protein.

How did I know? My body told me.

One week, in late November, I dreamed of eating chicken, every night. I'm not kidding. Each night, my mind created a surreal, Technicolor dream, informed by every part of my life. In the midst of it, the character that was me sat down amid the chaos to eat a plate of fried chicken. One night, I pulled apart a roasted chicken so fast that it stopped the motion of everything else around me. In my somnolent state, I was trying to tell myself something.

The next Saturday, my friend Gabe and I went out for Indian food at our favorite place just off 6th Street. We had been meeting there late at night, every few weeks, since the week we had both arrived in New York. Underneath a sea of Christmas lights tacked up on the ceiling, amid a blaze of sitar music, we usually ordered saag paneer and vegetarian curries with our mango lassis. Sometimes Gabe ordered a plate of tandoori chicken for himself, because this particular restaurant distinguished itself from the twenty-two other Indian places on the block by its fiery tandoori grill. Whenever that plate of smoky, red-charred chicken with the yogurt sauce arrived, Gabe grew quiet for a few moments as he gnawed at a piece. The Saturday night after the week full of chicken dreams, I looked at him eating, then reached my hand toward the tandoori chicken.

Gabe grabbed my hand. "What are you doing?" he looked at me in alarm.

"I want some chicken," I said plainly. And then I took a bite.

As he stared at me, amazed—for the six years he had known me, I had been a vegetarian—I tasted chicken for the first time in over a decade. The flesh slithered on my teeth. The juices roared along my tongue. The texture—ah, the ineffable texture—that nothing else had ever matched: solid, with softness, an indescribable yielding.

"Well?" Gabe asked, a little nervous.

I looked up at him, and then I wiped the sauce from my lips. "Could I have another piece?"

The next day, I ate a turkey sandwich for lunch.

I expected my body to revolt, but it didn't. Instead, I seemed to have unlocked the gate to a secret garden, and the grasses grew lusher by the day. My body desperately needed the protein, since I was probably malnourished in so many ways from having celiac disease. Even though I didn't have a name for it, I knew that something was askew. Listening to my body, closely, was important preparation for later days to come.

For a while, I stuck to eating only chicken or turkey, in sandwiches at coffee shops or roasted at the Cuban place across the street from me. However, when Thanksgiving loomed before me like the giant balloons bobbing along Central Park West, I decided to brave the winds and roast a turkey for my friends. Everyone praised its succulence. (I didn't cook it as long as my mother had.) To my surprise, I found the entire process—buying the meat and preparing it, watching it in the oven, and eating what I had made myself—satisfying, even rewarding. The next month, I roasted my first chicken.

For a few years, there was a quiet voice of guilt in the back of my mind about eating meat. After all, I thought I had been a better person by being a vegetarian. Priggish people sometimes found out that I had returned to my meat-eating ways and tried to lecture me over the dinner table. When I lived in London with the wealthy family, Madame could never seem to understand that I *had been* a vegetarian, instead of living it in the present tense. Because she was a vegetarian, she felt everyone should be one as well. One night, when she picked a fight with me, just before I decided to leave, she spat out: "And I hear you sometimes eat cold chicken in the kitchen at night!" By personifying the voice of moralistic horror in my head, she helped me to see how irrational I was being. My body wanted meat. I ate meat. There are other ways to live consciously.

When I returned to New York and wandered into the kitchen

to see one of my roommates—the one who had most loudly proclaimed the importance of *not eating meat*—hunched over a takeout chicken from down the street, I breathed a sigh of relief.

Back in my own life, I roasted chickens and sliced turkey breast for my sandwiches and baked fish for friends. Going to restaurants no longer meant studying the menus and interrogating the waiter about whether chicken stock had been used to flavor the soup. I just ordered the chicken or the fish. I still stayed away from any meat other than poultry. That seemed like too big a leap for a recent vegetarian to take. Beef? Too meaty. Pork? There must be a reason that religious people avoid it. Lamb? I had never eaten it. My mother didn't think it was safe, and I just thought of woolly little creatures gamboling in the grass. No. No real meat for me.

But once in a while, when I walked past the Metropolitan Museum on my way to a tutoring gig, my eyes stayed a beat longer than usual on the hot dog stand at the bottom of the steps. When I skated on 72nd Street, on my way to Central Park, I looked over at Gray's Papaya, the cheap hot dog stand that every New Yorker adored. Sharon and I had beers at the Corner Bistro after one of her comedy shows, and as she wolfed down one of their juicy burgers with caramelized onions, I watched her every bite. Slowly, I started to recognize what I had been feeling a few years before. I could hardly believe it, but it seemed my body wanted to eat red meat.

I carried that yearning with me when I went back home to Seattle in the summer of my brother's wedding. I stood on an enormous lawn, arm in arm with my brother. Those of us who were closest to him had spent the morning setting up the scene for the ceremony. It was near noon, and the guests were due in two hours. To thank us, Andy and his bride-to-be, Dana, were throwing a barbecue. Dana had quickly become one of my favorite people, and starting to know her that summer made me sad that I lived across the country. Solid, smart, and sure of herself, Dana was a compassionate veterinarian. She had a better understanding of animals than anyone I had ever met. A few weeks before, I had asked her why she wasn't a vegetarian, since she adored animals the way she did. She shrugged her shoulders. Ever pragmatic, she said, "You know, that's life. Our bodies are built to eat meat. I do." She had no guilt, no inner angst. She acted on what she felt.

So, that afternoon, moved and happy, feeling close, my brother and I stood on the site of his wedding, surveying the scene. He looked at the barbecues smoking, our friends eating, and said, "I'm sorry, Sis. There's nothing for you to eat. All we have is hamburgers and hot dogs." He put his arm around my shoulders to console me.

I looked at him, smelled the sweet acrid smoke of meat on the grill, and then said, "No problem. I'll have a hamburger."

"What!" he said, pulling away to see my face more clearly. He was as shocked as Gabe had been two years before. He knew that I had not eaten red meat in eighteen years.

"Seriously. I believe in taking what's offered. I want a burger."

He fetched me one, incredulous, then watched me bite into it. Is there any way to describe a hamburger, especially after eighteen years away from one? I can tell you these were nothing like the thin, frozen patties of my childhood. These were made with organic beef, which came from cows raised on the island, only five miles away from that site. My burger was thick, the insides a little pink, and the juices ran clear down my thumbs. That first taste is inextricably woven with the wedding, the return home, dancing on the lawn until the sun went down at ten, and a new feeling of peace within me.

The next day, I had another burger, this time on Julie's deck. Two days later, at Tita's house, I ate a steak, done rare. There was no going back now. I was no longer dipping my toes into the shallow waters. I had dived in.

Back in New York, I sat in a diner on 100th Street, with my dear friend Merida and our friend Will. Crammed into the red vinyl booths, the three of us sat talking about food. Will told us he was going to order the lamb chops. I admitted that I had never eaten lamb. Will was shocked. He had grown up in the South, where his family ate every kind of meat available. Merida looked a little horrified, maybe even a little disgusted. Her father had grown up in Ecuador, where she had spent nearly every summer, and she had stories about eating roasted guinea pig. I tried to evoke my image of little woolly creatures, but they just laughed at me. Lamb seemed like nothing to them. I wavered; I was curious. They urged me again. I relented. I took one bite, closed my eyes, and sighed. That lamb had the robust heft of beef, but it was more nuanced, a little chewier. Slightly sweeter. Not so demanding.

It makes me laugh, now, to think that I ate my first lamb in a diner, instead of at an expensive restaurant where the chef really knows how to cook it, tenderly. But life is full of contradictions.

Before I moved away from Manhattan, one of my last acts was to finally eat a hot dog from the stand in front of the Metropolitan Museum of Art. I lavished it with mustard and lingered before I bit into it. The squeak and chew, the pop of juices, the meaty texture along my tongue—every bite brought back memories of sitting in front of the television, watching my beloved Dodgers. I loved that hot dog.

Now, of course, I know that the bun would make me ill.

Why was I suddenly more comfortable eating meat, including the suspect processed ones, after more than a decade of feeling sanctimonious and scared of animal flesh? I think I had grown up. Now, please don't misunderstand me. We all have our reasons, and I have dear friends now who have been vegetarians and vegans all their lives. I respect them and feed them without any sense of judgment. By no means do I feel that being a vegetarian is a juvenile decision. However, for *me*, it was. I grew up with a mother who terrified me into thinking that beef cooked anything less than leathery could kill me, and a father who complied with all her wishes. Without my recognizing it, for years my mother's need for purity and safety, everything untainted and wrapped in cotton wool, was instilled in me, deeply. Hot dogs might have something unsavory in them? *Stay away.* But after I had moved away from my parents and had become

more comfortable with imperfections, through a meditation practice and living in Manhattan, I realized something. I wanted steak,
and I wanted it *rare*.

But I still didn't want to cook it.

Back in Seattle, I was teaching again, which gave me evenings to
cook, by myself and with friends. I still craved meat as much as I had
in New York, but I insisted that someone else make it for me.

The fact is that cooking meat intimidated me. After all, my role
models in the kitchen had burnt all our meat to the crisp edges. No
one had ever taught me how to cook a piece of meat with flavor.
Most of my friends had been vegetarians for years; even those who
were recovering vegetarians felt stymied by slabs of meat. Secretly,
I wished that I could be the kind of woman who could concoct a
succulent pot roast and feed a house full of people on a Sunday
afternoon. However, faced with three pounds of meat under plastic wrap, I lost my nerve and bought another package of chicken
breasts.

I needed a shot of courage.

Instead of finding the nerve to cook a pork tenderloin, I lost
consciousness on an early Sunday morning. Being T-boned by a
speeding car precluded the possibility of learning to grill T-bones
properly. The car accident in the dead of winter left me in terrible
pain for over a year. Opening my freezer during that time of my life
reminded me of my childhood: TV dinners, frozen spinach, and ice
cream treats. Beset by a pounding headache after I returned home
from school every day, I barely had the energy to cook. I opened
packages and ate pasta and bought pastries from the bakery down
the street from my new apartment. I felt lousy, all the time. Creating
homemade meals just felt like too much work. Cooking meat felt far
beyond my ken.

The next spring, for seven weeks, I could barely eat anything. I lay
on the couch, languishing away, bloated and infused with searing
pain. No one knew why. The doctors kept guessing, with the aid of

expensive tests. If I ate more than a tablespoon of food at a time, I felt as though my stomach would explode. And there were plenty of other ailments. When you're that ill, hunks of meat just don't appeal. Although I had always been a cheese hound, chèvre and Gouda fell out of favor, because anything with too much fat made me ache with pain. I won't even talk about the horrid morning of the avocado. So slowly, I winnowed my menu down to the foods that seemed to go down easy. Crackers, homemade white loaves from my friend Mary, Popsicles, canned chicken noodle soup, and ginger ale.

With the exception of the ginger ale, everything I ate, one tablespoon at a time, contained gluten. That is why I was so sick.

When I finally did have the answer and stopped eating gluten, I felt enormously better almost immediately. But by this time, my small intestines were damaged rather badly. You see, celiac disease means that my body reads gluten as a toxin and thus sends out fierce antibodies to attack it when it enters my system. Since patches of the villi had been flattened by my own antibodies, my small intestines were no longer capable of producing the enzyme necessary to digest lactose. This is why people with full-blown, active celiac disease become lactose intolerant by proxy. In fact, from what I have come to understand, some people realize they have celiac disease because they suddenly can no longer digest cheese or milk.

In order to heal from celiac disease, I only had to eat great, gluten-free food. I haven't taken any drugs or endured any surgeries. Instead, the body heals itself. After six months to a year of completely avoiding gluten, I have healthy intestines, as though none of this has ever happened. Years of damage simply disappeared.

But for the first couple months after my diagnosis, I didn't eat anything involving meat or dairy. Meat just felt too hard to digest, and dairy just didn't go over well. I put aside the beef and brie. I had been feeling rotten for so long that I happily avoided both, just happy to be eating and feeling the physical pangs of hunger again. First, I focused on the foods that happen to not contain meat or dairy: warm spinach salads, crisp carrots with a wonderful crunch, broiled tofu with peanut sauce, and juicy watermelon on a hot summer's day. The broad red bowl on my chrome kitchen shelves was perpetually filled with fresh produce. My kitchen table was almost always mounded with herbs, vegetables ready to be chopped, and fruit just begging to be made into crumbles and sorbets.

So, for about two months, I was a gluten-free vegan.

Being a vegetarian for all those years was inadvertently great preparation for having to eat gluten-free. I already knew what it was like to wander my way through the maze of the day while trying to avoid certain foods. I already knew how to ask questions about ingredients and to choose the best restaurants. I had switched the food I cannot eat, this time because of the direct consequences on my health. I am choosing my own way.

All my attitudes toward food shifted once I realized I could not eat gluten. A certain girlish squeamishness about cooking meat disappeared as soon as I realized I would never eat a steak again unless I learned to sear it myself. At the time, I was overwhelmed by the sudden knowledge of all the places that gluten can hide, as well as the dangers of cross-contamination. It all felt so flummoxing. My first response to these changes was to stay at home and learn to cook.

It was time to dive in. No more staying on the edges of cooking meat with an endless array of chicken breast recipes and fish several times a week. When my hunger returned, it roared in me. When my intestines healed, I craved more protein. Everything in my life had guided me to this point.

For the first time in my life, paradoxically, I found I had no fear of food. I didn't stay away from healthy fats like olive oil and nuts because they might have too many calories. I didn't count the number of bites I took per day. I no longer skirted the edges of skirt steaks. After a lifetime of feeling lousy and being undernourished, I saw the food available to me as a chance to eat well.

Other than not eating gluten, I restricted myself from nothing. As long as it was fresh and whole and in season, I ate it. I opened my arms to great food. Finally, I ate without guilt. No residual feeling of being a bad person lingered within me if I seared some pork chops.

I was feeding myself. I was healing. And I learned to play. Because I was cooking for myself as a way of ensuring that my body was well fed, instead of cooking to impress with the grandeur of my recipes, I was not afraid of making mistakes. If I threw a steak into the oven, and it crisped up too much, I realized that I just needed to cook it a little less the next time. Even the ground beef I cooked for casseroles no longer brought up resonances of all those evenings at home, standing in front of the stove while my parents fought in the living room. Instead, I was feeding myself. And I was determined to live well.

Eating well meant eating meat, at least for me.

Of course, it helps to have a good butcher. Once I started living gluten-free, I realized how lucky I was to have three independent businesses within five miles of me, all three offering some of the best meats and seafood available in Seattle. Not one of them has a decór that has been updated in the last twenty years. Not one of them is a chain. They all feed me well.

A&J Meats is located about 150 yards from my front door. When I walk into the wood-paneled room with glass display cases, I feel as if I have walked into a butcher shop from the 1950s. The tops of the cases are lined with bottles of locally made tartar sauce, barbecue spices in tins, and an old-fashioned ticket dispenser for the customers who throng into the place. Milling about the store are neighborhood moms and dads, their toddlers running toward the hot dogs. If it is Saturday morning, then a woman in her eighties comes in for a single lamb chop; she is given preferential treatment, because she has been a customer at the shop for longer than most of the butchers have been working there. Behind the counters walk friendly men and women in crisp white aprons, ready with smiles and advice. I ask my favorite butchers—one of whom is a woman—what is good that day. This curiosity and trust led me to cook my first flank steak, pork tenderloin, and duck breast. Every time, the butchers walked me through the process of searing or roasting, both with their handouts copied on colored paper and their murmured words of encouragement. Even if the meat shrink-wrapped in supermarkets is slightly cheaper, the personal service I receive at A&J's is worth the extra cost.

When I am down at Pike Place Market, which is at least once a week, I walk past the loud and showy stall where young guys in orange overalls toss fish above the tourists' heads. Tucked behind it is Don and Joe's, a little triangular butcher's stall. The men behind these glass cases have chapped hands and calloused fingers. Every one of them has a blue-inked tattoo on his upper arm and a baseball cap pulled low over his eyes. It has nothing of the polished gleam of Whole Foods or the fluorescent lighting of Safeway. Instead, Don and Joe's feels real. Those men are at home behind those cases, and they know their meat. Don and Joe's offers spectacular applewood-smoked bacon and free-range eggs grown on a farm thirty miles from that spot. I still haven't tried the lamb tongue, however, even though I do admit the tongues have a certain symmetry all lined up in the case.

When I want fresh seafood, served without any pretension, I drive over to University Seafood Market. Dale greets me with a lopsided grin. He reaches into the case full of fish with a gnarled hand, and then brings up a filet of petrale sole for me. One day, I will wander from my now-familiar fish selections and take a chance on the opa. His father owned the store—opened sixty years before—where Dale began working as a teenager. Now he runs the front, and his savvy wife, Jeannette, handles all the billing in back. I'm fairly sure that each of the other five employees there has worked at University Seafood for over twenty years. In fact, they have all worked so long together that they are starting to look the same: bushy moustaches, smudgy eyeglasses, and well-used hands. Those hands reach for game hens or pigeon, and my mind starts racing with the possibilities of a food I have never cooked before. One of my friends, a wonderful woman in her seventies who ran a French restaurant in Seattle in the 1980s, says she will only buy her duck fat at University Seafood. It's easy to see why. Even though the space is tiny—about six customers can fit in its confines at once—and the walls are festooned with old newspaper stories, fish netting, and pictures from the 1940s, this place offers the most personal service I have ever found from a seafood market. On top of that, every time I am in there, a chef from a local restaurant is in, signing an invoice and carrying out boxes of black cod for that night's specials.

We never shopped at stores like these when I was a kid. We went to Alpha-Beta and Vons, huge fluorescent-lit emporiums of food. The meat we ate sat wrapped in plastic, sanitized, far removed from the animal from which it came. Eating that meat felt entirely anonymous, disconnected from the world. Now, however, I feel part of the process of buying food that becomes part of my body. Now I want to know from what part of the world—and from what part of the animal—my meat and seafood comes. I never go to the grocery store to buy beef anymore. Instead, I walk into A&J's and ask for grass-fed tenderloin, grow in western Washington, from a farm that treats its cows well. The guys at University Seafood buy their food from only the most reputable sources, people they trust. Most of the time, they are buying directly from the fishermen, who have been up in the wild waters of Alaska trolling for salmon just days before.

Every year, I am privileged to teach at a fine arts camp in Sitka, Alaska. Two of my favorite students there are sisters, buoyant and open, alive and ridiculous. Their father is a commercial fisherman. During the summer, in salmon season, he is gone for days to weeks at a time, coming into harbor only when his boat is filled with fresh fish. After he delivers the salmon to the processing plant, where they are sent to Seattle and beyond, he goes out again. One summer, Berett and Adrienne invited me over to their home for dinner. Their mother—just as feisty and funny as her daughters—handed me a plate of barbecued salmon, the remaining portion of the fish her husband had caught the day before. In fact, she told me, when she woke up that morning, she found a black plastic garbage bag on the porch, with a tail fin sticking out the top. Her husband had hand-delivered a salmon for our dinner, in the early-morning hour he had spent on shore before returning to the boat again.

Need I say that it was the most delicious salmon I have ever eaten in my life?

Recently, there has been a movement to label certain fish "organic." Now, I am a huge fan of organic foods, particularly in vegetables and fruits. However, wild Alaskan salmon, or sablefish, or halibut, will never be labeled organic, because it is not grown under conditions that can be regulated. Instead, Berett and Adrienne's father pulls those fish from the deep waters off his home. Farmed fish can be managed and watched, but it is not as good as wild salmon. "Organic" fish is a misnomer, the kind of scare tactic that my mother would have followed if she were raising us now.

The father of those girls has a hard-working life. But he loves it. His father was a fisherman, and he chose the life of the open sea instead of something a little safer. All over Sitka, on the back bumpers of trucks, bright red stickers proclaim: FRIENDS DON'T LET FRIENDS EAT FARMED FISH. Sure, farmed fish may seem more abundant in the grocery stores, and it may be a little less expensive to buy. But the next time you reach for a piece of it, remember Berett and Adrienne's father. Remember, as well, that eating wild Alaskan salmon is better for the environment and for your body than farmed salmon could ever be.

The more consciously we eat our food, the better fed we are.

After having lived as a vegetarian for much of my life, I respect the choice. But I have to say—if you are flirting with the idea of eating meat, especially if you have gone gluten-free and are worried about having so many foods restricted from your diet—the following recipes might just tempt you. Who knows what you might discover?

juicy burgers

One October, my dear friend Cindy came to visit me in Seattle. Cindy bubbles with ebullience for life in every conversation. No one can doubt when we are in the same room together—or even in the same city—for all the loud laughter and endless explosions of agreement. Most of our conversations revolve around food. She was impressed with everything we ate that weekend. But neither one of us could believe our food luck when we ate the lamb burger at Café Campagne. It was the juiciest burger I had ever eaten, but it was more than that. Almost every burger I had ever eaten, even the great ones, tasted like a big hunk of burger. This burger had layers of taste I had never experienced before. A little rosemary, a nibble of garlic, some dash of a succulence I could not name. Every bite tasted slightly different from the one before. Cindy and I stared at each other across the table, astonished. We still talk about it, three years later.

Once I went gluten-free, however, it seemed I would live on only the memory of that burger. Eating a burger in a restaurant seemed impossible. Some restaurants use bread crumbs in their burgers. Nope. What was a burger without a good bun? That was right out. It became impossible to find a place where I could eat french fries, even if I did order a plain burger without a bun. Almost every restaurant in America fries its potatoes in the same fryer as its onion rings or crab cakes or fried desserts. That cross-contamination would make me sick. Thus, what choice was I facing? A beef patty without a bun.

I made up my own burger. Remembering that lamb burger at Café Campagne, I came up with this concoction. It doesn't really need a bun—although there are some good commercial gluten-free mixes on the market—because it will stay in your mind on its own.

A Juicy Burger

1 pound ground sirloin
1 tablespoon Worcestershire sauce (gluten-free)
2 teaspoons mixed fresh herbs: rosemary, thyme, parsley
1 teaspoon minced garlic
1 teaspoon kosher salt
1 teaspoon cracked black pepper

Preheating. Preheat the oven to 450 degrees F.

Mixing the patties. Mix all the ingredients together with your hands and form two thick patties.

Pan-searing the burgers. Heat a sauté pan over high heat. When it is hot, sear each patty on one side until browned—2 to 3 minutes. Turn over the patties and put the sauté pan into the oven.

Finishing the burgers. Cook for 5 to 7 minutes, or until the internal temperature of the hamburgers has reached 145 degrees F on your meat thermometer. (This is for a medium-rare burger.) Remove the patties from the oven and eat them the way you like to eat hamburgers.

Feeds 2.

inspiration at the IACP

One day in March, I stood in the Washington State convention center, smiling so hard I thought the top of my head might fall off.

That year, the convention for the International Association for Culinary Professionals (IACP) happened to be in Seattle. There was no way I'd pass up the opportunity to be around people who cook, take photographs of, and write about food. They might as well have named the event SIOH: Shauna's Idea of Heaven.

The next few days felt like a bonanza of classes, shaking hands, sampling foods, and being given free stuff. I took hours of classes on food writing, how to make a career out of food, how to use the five senses to describe the food we eat, the art of the food memoir, and the politics of food. After the third hour-and-a-half-long seminar of the day (and especially on the third day in a row of this), I thought I would be enervated and squirming. Nope. I was the student sitting forward on her chair, vigorously nodding, awake without coffee, writing it all down. I dread faculty meetings and education conferences; I'm usually the student at the back writing scurrilous notes about the drone in the room. But at the IACP convention, I just couldn't get enough of it.

I made a mental note of that, as well. Was teaching right for me?

The highlight was a gala evening at Pike Place Market, with fourteen hundred people stuffed into the long hallways, surging around the stalls, plastic cups of wine in hand, standing close and talking fast. Behind every low table—filled during the day with arts and crafts—stood one of the top chefs of Seattle, cooking spectacular food on small burners. Tom Douglas danced around woks, making Szechuan salt-and-pepper prawns for people. The chef from Cascadia offered vodka-infused salmon with Douglas fir syrup and the top of a fiddlehead fern. The chefs at Crush handed out freshly made s'mores with marshmallows and graham crackers made from scratch. (They were kind enough to make me a s'more without the graham cracker.) From the Herbfarm, perhaps the best restaurant in Washington State, was offered cinnamon-basil ice cream. I was happy and well fed.

I started to realize, with an increasing urgency, that I was in the right place. Waking up early had felt like a joy, instead of the drudge of early-morning alarms for school. I could feel a shift happening, in my gut.

The best part of all this—as always for me—was meeting the people. I met more alive, interesting people in one place than I had ever met before. Some of my favorites were fellow food bloggers. The inimitable David Lebovitz—who brought me delectable chocolates from France—was a constant source of amazement. Sweet and tart both, he made the best breakfast companion I've had in a long time.

So, in essence, I learned one lesson over and over again at this conference: food people equals good people.

I left the IACP conference with bags stuffed full of goodies and my head stuffed full of ideas. My spirits had been raised and my food sensibilities elevated. When I dove into the bag full of goodies the following week, I found hilarious items, including the pork chop–shaped mousepad I had won by correctly guessing where the tenderloin was located on a large-scale drawing of a pig. I couldn't resist putting it by the computer, to remind me. It sits there still.

That absurdly funny prize—and the innovative ideas of the chefs and writers I encountered—somehow inspired this pork recipe.

Barbecued Pork with Aromatic Jasmine Rice

1 cup ketchup
1 cup rice wine vinegar
1 cup oyster sauce (gluten-free)
5 garlic cloves, peeled and smashed
½ bunch green onions, sliced thin
1 cup jasmine rice
1½ cups water
½ stalk lemongrass, bruised
1 tablespoon unsalted butter
1 small nub of fresh ginger, peeled and chopped in large chunks
¼ cup thinly sliced white onions
1 teaspoon kosher salt
1 teaspoon cracked black pepper
1 pork tenderloin, about 1½ pounds
1 teaspoon kosher salt
½ teaspoon white pepper

Preheating. Preheat the oven to 450 degrees F.

Making the barbecue sauce. In a saucepan, bring the ketchup, rice wine vinegar, oyster sauce, garlic cloves, and green onions to a boil over medium-high heat. Turn the heat down to medium and let the sauce simmer for 30 minutes, stirring occasionally. Strain the barbecue sauce and set it aside.

Preparing the rice. Put the rice, water, lemongrass, butter, ginger, white onions, salt, and pepper into another saucepan on the stove and bring the mixture to a boil. Reduce to medium-low heat and cover tightly. Simmer for about 20 minutes, or until all the water has been absorbed. Do not stir the rice while it is cooking. Allow the rice to stand, off the burner, for 5 to 10 minutes, while you are preparing the pork.

Roasting the pork. Heat a sauté pan over high heat. Season the tenderloin with salt and pepper and sear it on all sides in the hot pan. When the tenderloin is seared, put the pan in the preheated oven and let it cook for 5 minutes. Take the pan from the oven, remove the tenderloin for a moment, and strain the grease from the pan. Add a cup of the barbecue sauce to the tenderloin and let it cook for 3 minutes more.

Serving the dish. Slice up the pork and lay over a small mound of the aromatic rice. Pour the remaining barbecue sauce over the pork.

Feeds 2.

salmon in the spring

There is something rich, with unexpected depth, about a great piece of salmon. I feel as though I am eating the Pacific Northwest—the green trees, the briny sea, the wind in January, the blue skies of August, the Olympic Mountains at sunset—whenever I eat salmon.

In late May, a year after my celiac diagnosis, I met Tara, one of my favorite food bloggers, from San Francisco. She and I had begun writing months before, because she had found my Web site in the midst of following a gluten-free diet. After long, enthusiastic letters back and forth, she decided to start her own food blog. A writer and an editor, Tara wanted to test the waters of food writing. Within a couple of months, her blog, Tea and Cookies, was considered one of the best-written food sites on the Internet.

By the time we finally met in person, she and I had written so many e-mails to each other and had left so many comments on each other's sites that we felt as though we knew each other well. I invited her into my home before I physically met her.

When I opened the door, there she was, just as I had expected her—smiling wide and starting to talk already. We picked up the conversation where we had left off in e-mails, and we naturally gravitated toward the kitchen. Within moments, we had our hands in the food together.

For part of our multicourse lunch, I seared us a couple pieces of wild Alaskan salmon, just come into season. A chef I had met recently had given me the secret to cooking salmon well: serve it rare. It's funny that I had long ago given up my parents' way of charcoaling all meat to the core, but I had continued to cook my fish until it was dry. At the same time, I was a sushi hound; I ate raw fish with delight. This time, I seared the salmon in a skillet for a minute, then threw it into the hot oven and cooked it for just a few moments. All the while, I was talking with Tara.

When I laid it in front of Tara, she looked a little stunned. Her face softened into a smile, and then she took a bite. After she had finished—quite rapidly—she said to me, "You know, I don't really like fish."

"Wait!" I exclaimed. "Why didn't you tell me before I started cooking it?"

"I didn't want to be rude," she said. "But listen—I really like this salmon."

She explained that she had been raised a vegetarian and had only recently started dabbling in meat and fish. No one had ever cooked fish like this before. She said, "I guess I'm going to have to change my mind about fish."

It really isn't the stunning recipe that makes for great food. It's just paying attention and figuring out how to do it well. That's all it takes to make someone else happy with food, and start off a wonderful friendship right.

Pan-Seared Salmon

½ teaspoon kosher salt
½ teaspoon cracked black pepper
2 fillets wild Alaskan salmon, skinned
2 tablespoons high-quality olive oil

Preparing. Preheat the oven to 500 degrees F. Season the salmon fillets with salt and pepper and set aside.

Pan-searing the salmon. Heat a sauté pan over high heat. (You will know it is hot enough when you can put a small drop of water on the surface of the pan and the water evaporates immediately.) Add the olive oil. When the oil is hot enough to move around the pan easily, add the salmon, fleshy side down. Cook for 1 to 2 minutes, or until browned.

Finishing the salmon. Put the pan in the oven and let the salmon cook until the internal temperature is 120 degrees F as registered on a meat thermometer. That is medium-rare, and it will be delicious.

Suggestion. This will work for any fish you wish you to cook.

Feeds 2.

6

going against the grain

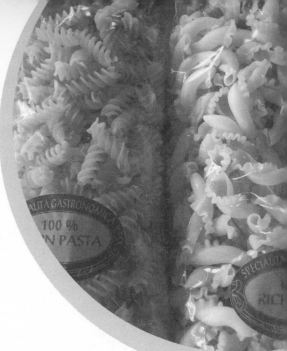

When my little brother was in the third grade, he grew constipated. I don't mean one-day constipated. I mean three-months constipated. Constipated to the point that my parents took him to our family doctor, who prescribed him enemas. My brother was only eight years old. He was such a sensitive little guy that it disturbed him when the substitute teacher did math in the wrong part of the day. The dingy bathrooms at school didn't have doors on the stalls, at least for the boys, and my little brother couldn't tolerate the lack of privacy. So, he didn't go. Of course, there were the trials and tribulations at home, which might have contributed to the stoppage.

It might also have helped if we had ever eaten grains.

I don't think I ever ate a whole grain of anything when I was growing up. By the time it reached my lips, every grain had been pummeled, sugared, and packaged. Bread was white and airy-doughy, wrapped in a plastic covering. Most crackers were flat in taste and white in color, flecked with salt, missing nutrition. Even rice—always white—had been stripped of its nutrients and slipped into plastic bags with holes for boiling in a minute.

Breakfast is the best chance to start the day right. Eat a bowl of something packed with vitamins and fiber, and you'll be walking well all day. What did we eat as kids? Sugary cereals that floated in a bowl of milk, which sometimes turned a sickly pink from all the food dyes present in the package. Certainly, hot cereal would have served us better, but the oatmeal we ate came in little packets with lumps of brown sugar already injected.

Maybe we were always constipated.

When I was a bit older, my parents decided to have a party around the pool. They arranged little taquitos they had reheated from the freezer. Guacamole from the store with greasy corn chips. Onion dip and potato chips. And some soft Monterey Jack cheese with little shreds of red-dyed chiles. As the party approached, my mother realized she didn't have any crackers. In a panic, she sent my father to the store. I'm sure she wanted something standard, like overly crisp Wheat Thins or even the daringly grainy Triscuits. Instead, he came home with a giant red-and-white package of crackers. They weren't Saltines, but a cheaper version, made in Mexico. He had grabbed them because they were the least expensive one on the shelf. When my mother turned over the package, she read on the bottom, stamped in bold letters: FIT FOR HUMAN CONSUMPTION. This sent her into a tizzy. According to my mother, if a company has to reassure you that the crackers you're holding are okay for you to eat, you probably should watch out. She sent my father back to the store for some familiar crackers.

We still laugh about it today. But now I'm laughing for different reasons.

Today, America is in the midst of a whole-grain crisis. We just don't eat them. Nutritionists and the U.S. Department of Agriculture recommend that everyone eat at least three servings of whole grains a day. What does that mean? Usually, one serving is defined as half an ounce of whole grains. That's five whole-grain crackers or one slice of whole-grain bread or three cups of popcorn. That shouldn't be too hard to eat in a day, should it? Well, for most Americans, it seems impossible. The average American eats only one serving of whole grains per day. Because multinational food companies are advertising some of their foods as containing whole grains, many people think they are getting their one serving a day from a big handful of cheese puffs. Worse yet, 30 percent of Americans never eat a whole grain. Not once. All year.

Apparently, my family was not the only one constipated.

A cursory look at medical sites on the Internet or books about health, one conversation with a nutritionist, or just gut instinct tells us that we should eat whole grains. They're good for us. Eating the proper amount of whole grains can reduce cholesterol dramatically. This lessens the risk of heart disease. Numerous studies have shown that people who eat whole grains are at lower risk for diabetes and various cancers. B vitamins, iron, magnesium, selenium—you name it, whole grains have it. Without doubt, whole grains are full of good-for-you nutrition.

Also, whole grains fill you up and leave you feeling satisfied. Have you ever eaten a big bowl of hot cereal for breakfast, then felt hungry half an hour later? Probably not. That's because the fiber in whole-grain cereals takes longer to digest than other, simpler foods, which means your body waits longer to decide you need to eat again. Eat whole grains daily, and you might not eat as much.

Besides, whole grains help you poop.

Whole grains and other sources of dietary fiber do not break down in the bowels the way other foods do, since they are insoluble. That means they cannot be dissolved by water, which is also floating around in there. Some part of that fiber is left, undigested. As the fiber moves through the system, it pulls water and other foods with it, like a pied piper of poop. This is how your body creates a cohesive bowel movement, the kind that leaves you feeling satisfied and healthy.

There's no other way around it—everybody poops. But we're afraid to talk about that bodily function in this country. We have been trained to believe that it's rude. Some of you may have been shocked to read the previous paragraph. But it's a fact that we need to poop, and poop well. When I was deathly ill with celiac disease, I knew something was terribly wrong from the fact that I was as constipated as my little brother had been decades before. Nothing was passing. I was all stopped up.

Bowel movements are one of the best indicators of health in a human being. It wasn't until after I was diagnosed with celiac disease that I realized I had been either constipated or having diarrhea all my life. It was the rare day when I experienced a bowel movement without some struggle or surprise. That's what a lifetime of eating processed foods, microwave meals, and fast foods on the run will do to you. For decades, I thought that's what it meant to be alive. Since Americans are eating so many foods stripped of nutrition—and the closest we come to healthy eating is using "enriched" white flour— our bodies have forgotten how to digest.

Years ago, a trainer at a gym advised me to eat quinoa. I had never heard of the stuff, and when I went to the local chain grocery store, the teenage clerk looked at me askance when I asked for it. I had to venture into a health food store. Dubious at first of something I did not know, I grew to love the grain, with its delicate, nutty flavor. I began substituting it for my rice in the evenings. On the nights I ate some lean meat, a few vegetables, and steamed quinoa, I went to bed feeling mysteriously better.

That's because there had been no gluten in that meal.

Over time, I even developed a taste for the oatmeal I made on the stove, steel-cut and made slowly instead of ripped from a little packet and ready in a minute. In the last few years before my celiac diagnosis, when I sensed that I needed to eat more healthfully, I ate oatmeal for breakfast every morning. Topped with blueberries or roasted hazelnuts, oatmeal filled me up and set me on my day far more sturdily than sugary cereals ever could.

How could I know that the oatmeal was also making me sick? When I found out I had celiac disease, I was open to throwing out the wheat, rye, and barley immediately. But could I live without my oatmeal? Those who must eat gluten-free are also advised to avoid oats. Inherently, oats are gluten-free, but the process by which most oats are produced in the United States—on an assembly line still coated with flour from the product before it and thus cross-contaminating the oats—makes them suspect for those with celiac disease. Reluctantly, I gave up my oatmeal, knowing that it would make me healthier.

What was I to do? There I was, a woman determined to eat more whole grains per day than the majority of Americans, and I was told I could not eat the most familiar grains in my repertoire. I had visions of living on Metamucil for the rest of my life.

What a gift a bit of structure can be. Because I knew that I would have to work to eat enough grains, and because I was stubborn enough to not want to give up my baking altogether, I began investigating gluten-free grains. Over the next few months, I found grains that I had never heard of before, grains that I have come to love far more than wheat.

Having enjoyed so many Ethiopian meals with friends, and especially the injera bread made with teff, I started to experiment with the naturally gluten-free flour at home. I created a roasted red pepper and sweet corn quiche with a teff flour crust, the crust silky soft and that essential taste of summer singing out.

Next, I discovered amaranth, a grain whose name I only dimly knew. I began toasting amaranth in a scorching hot skillet, watching the tiny grains the size of poppy seeds darken and dance. After they had finished popping, I ate them with organic milk and maple syrup, for a winter breakfast cereal. The roasted corn smell of the toasted amaranth filled the house all day with its enveloping warmth.

Prior to my celiac diagnosis, millet had appeared before me only as seed at the bottom of a friend's birdcage. Once I learned that the grain is gluten-free and filled with nutrition, I started experimenting with it. Toasted, millet is crunchy with a soft bite, and I started combining it with chickpeas and spinach for a warm grains salad.

I returned to quinoa, simmering it with a wild mushroom stock, and then topping it with roasted yellow peppers, flash-sautéed green beans, and cumin carrot slivers. I threw together a summer quinoa tabouleh, with slow-roasted tomatoes, fresh cucumbers, tomato vinegar, and tiny wedges of locally grown goat cheese.

Want to come over for dinner?

Rice, of course, yielded creamy mushroom risottos, vivid stir-fries with twelve different slivered vegetables—flavored with ume plum vinegar and wheat-free tamari—and sweet rice flour for baking chewy almond cookies.

I experimented with sorghum flour, learning how to make my own rotis, puffed thin and crunchy, like the ones I eat in my favorite Indian restaurants. Later, I learned to add it to my bread recipes, which gave olive loaves depth and a softness like focaccia.

And this is deprivation?

I never feel deprived on a gluten-free diet. How could I, with these gorgeous, gluten-free foods to sustain me? Eventually, I started to think, "Gluten is the most boring food in the world."

Eat some of these grains regularly, and I think you might agree with me.

amaranth

As a kid, I was completely out of touch with the way food was actually made. Everything arrived in such a state that the manufacturers might have already chewed it for me. Polystyrene, plastic, cardboard—those were the substances I knew. I never knew that I could enjoy eating food in its whole state. Or that a weed that grows on the side of the road could turn out to be one of my favorite grains.

A few months after going gluten-free, I was walking through a Seattle farmers' market with a friend. July sunshine spilled on our shoulders. Everything felt expansive. The organic fruits and vegetables displayed on the tables enticed me to try them. I walked by a stand selling greens I had never seen before. They were leafy green like spinach, but thinner, more ornate. In the middle of each leaf was a burst of purple. Three stalls down was another pile of the unusual greens. Clearly, Chinese spinach had come into season that week. Fascinated, I asked the young girl behind the table where these came from, originally. She shrugged her shoulders. After handing her a dollar bill, I took the greens home, determined to find out.

Thank goodness for the Internet. After a bit of searching, I was able to locate a photograph of Chinese spinach almost immediately. When I started reading, I was even more excited. Amaranth? "Chinese spinach" is actually the leaves of one species of the amaranth plant, the same plant that produces the gluten-free grain I had most been wanting to try.

Amaranth was first grown domestically seven thousand years ago in Mexico. For the Aztecs, it was a sacred grain, used in almost every aspect of their lives. Historians believe that amaranth was as important as maize to the Aztecs, who used it to feed themselves and their animals and in their blood sacrifices. The conquistadores claimed that the Aztecs used amaranth in ritualistic killings, mixing amaranth, lime, and blood to form little idols that would be eaten in the middle of ceremonies. Is this true? We'll never know for sure. And it's not clear if the conquistadores made it a crime to grow amaranth or simply looked down upon it. Clearly, they didn't approve, because amaranth nearly disappeared forever over the next century. If it hadn't been grown secretly on farms high on the Andes or in hidden pockets of Mexico, amaranth would no longer exist in the world.

I'm glad that it does.

Amaranth is eaten all over the world, especially in some of the poorer places. In Nepal, people mill amaranth flour to make little cakes, which they eat daily. People in Peru have learned how to make beer out of amaranth, called *chichi*. And in Ecuador, women drink a distilled liquid of amaranth grain to regulate their menstrual cycle. It is easy to produce prolific crops of amaranth—each plant can produce forty thousand to sixty thousand seeds, making it an economically efficient crop. Amaranth is high in iron and fiber, as well as being packed with amino acids such as lysine, making it full of important proteins.

No wonder the National Academy of Sciences recommended the commercial cultivation of amaranth in the United States, at a conference on ancient foods, in the early 1980s. This relatively recent recommendation has meant that most Americans have not heard of amaranth.

Those interested in whole grains decades before they became trendy, however, knew about amaranth. When I told my friend Tita that I was experimenting with amaranth recipes, she laughed and said: "Oh, amaranth. Everyone was making bread out of that in the seventies. It grew like weeds where I lived." Of course, she grew up in Madison, Wisconsin, in the 1960s. She was a hippie.

Now, after going gluten-free, I have learned to cultivate a friendly relationship with amaranth as well. Amaranth has a light, nutty taste, with a smell like roasted corn. The flour makes an excellent crepe, an outstanding cake (when mixed with other gluten-free flours, like rice), and a healthy muffin with spiced pumpkin and ground flax-seed. I've even learned how to make whole-grain crackers with it, which are—of course—fit for human consumption.

a new breakfast cereal

After going gluten-free, I was bereft of my sugary kid smacks and my adult oatmeal. What was I to do for breakfast cereal? Always on the lookout for a whole-grain breakfast, one day I turned on the stove and waited for my skillet to heat up almost to the point of scorching. When it grew so hot I thought I'd set off the smoke alarm the next minute, I threw in tiny amaranth seeds and waited to see what would happen. I didn't have to wait long. They began popping, jumping off the skillet, dancing, and fluttering. The smell that wafted to my nose made me pop a little, too. It smelled a bit like popcorn, with more warmth, a little more depth. The grains were toasted a dark brown, a tiny bit plumper. The entire kitchen smelled of roasted amaranth. I couldn't wait to eat it.

I find that I love foods that make me feel as if I'm playing, like a kid, when I cook it. And this is definitely one of them.

I spooned the hot grains into my favorite red bowl, filled it with heated milk, a tablespoon of maple syrup, and a few spoonfuls of homemade blackberry jam. And I ate.

Ah, the decadence. It doesn't taste like anything else. I can feel the little seeds in my mouth, crunchy and mushy at the same time. Easy going down, but quite clearly a whole grain, as well. And all morning, afterward, I felt energized and clean.

Now, I eat it for breakfast once a week.

I don't miss Count Chocula at all anymore.

Popped Amaranth Cereal

¼ cup organic amaranth seeds
½ cup warm milk
½ teaspoon cinnamon
½ teaspoon ground ginger
1 tablespoon organic cane sugar
¼ cup chopped dates
2 tablespoons chopped pecans

Popping the amaranth. Bring a skillet to heat over high heat. When the skillet is so hot that beads of water can dance across it, toss in the amaranth seeds. As soon as the seeds begin popping—like miniature popcorn kernels—stir them continuously with a wooden spoon for about 5 minutes. When most of the seeds have turned darker brown and plump, just before they burn, take the skillet off the heat and put the popped amaranth into a bowl.

Making the cereal. Pour the warm milk over the popped amaranth. Add the cinnamon, ginger, and sugar, and stir. Top with the chopped dates and pecans.

Feeds 1.

millet

I remember thick, syrupy-sweet chocolate sauce, poured from a can; processed cheese food; soft white bread; mushy tomatoes; and crisp little chocolate-chip cookies, tumbling into a bowl, disguised as breakfast cereal.

Almost all the tastes of my childhood were cloying, muddled into one, even suffocating. With everything packaged for convenience, the food of my childhood fooled me into thinking that everything tasted sickly sweet or overly salty. For years, I did not know what food truly tasted like.

Of course, without ever eating whole grains, how could I know how much I'd enjoy the clean, simple tastes of something like millet?

Mild and light, little beads of millet have a subtly nuanced sweetness. When I boil them with chicken stock, they emerge golden and creamy. The adaptable millet grain takes on the flavor of whatever it contacts, but it still maintains its clean, clear essence.

Millet was first grown in China, where it was revered for thousands of years as one of the country's five most sacred grains. (Its name in Chinese—*xiaomi*—translates to "little rice.") Millet also grew across the Roman empire in its heyday. However, as is true for most of the gluten-free grains, millet somehow fell out of favor with the upper classes. Today, millet is regarded as poor man's food throughout much of the world, including the United States, where it is mostly sold as bird feed.

Millet actually has more iron than any other grain besides teff. It makes a complete protein and cooks up wonderfully well. Farmers in the Midwest grow it in abundance. But I had never heard of it until I had to go gluten-free. Since then, I've eaten millet at least once a week. Mixed in soups, it's slightly nutty, with a soft bite. I adore it with any kind of beans but especially pinto and fava beans. Sometimes, I simply cook it with mushroom stock and cumin, then garnish it with handfuls of Italian parsley. Millet flour gives gluten-free baked goods a crumbly texture, which is why I like to fold it into zucchini breads and chocolate-chip cookies.

Who *needs* regular flour? With grains like millet, I've started to prefer the alternative instead of longing for what I once knew. After all, this one tastes good, and it won't make me sick.

Most of my best food experiences come from random happenstance, it seems.

One day, while I was buying my daily coffee at the shop where I sit in the corner and write for hours, I talked to my favorite barista about her lunch. She exulted over the jicama she had eaten, along with fresh fruit. Jicama . . .

My brain caught upon it, the idea of that crisp, delicious white tuber, cut into strips.

By the time I had walked to my table, I had an idea. I looked it up in one of my favorite books about food. Jicama goes well with chiles and lime? Hmm. When I left the coffee shop, I had a new recipe in mind. Time to go to the store.

There's always a tug at the back of my brain when a new food idea enters. Something stops. For a moment, I seize. My gut says yes. And then my mind won't let go. I walk around for a few moments like a zombie, chanting in my head, "Jicama. Jicama." Finally, I have to go do something about it, just to move onto something new. . . . Like create a dish like this.

Chilled Millet Salad with Jicama and Mango

4 jalapeño peppers
2 cups water
1 cup millet
2 teaspoons butter
1 teaspoon kosher salt
1 ripe mango
1 medium-size jicama (about as big as your fist)
juice of 2 limes
1 avocado
1 teaspoon cayenne pepper

Roasting the jalapeño peppers. Preheat the oven to 500 degrees F. Place the jalapeño peppers in a baking pan, coat them with a little olive oil, and put the pan in the oven. After 5 minutes or so, take the pan out of the oven and turn the peppers with tongs. Put the pan back in and let the peppers' skin char, somewhat. This should take about 20 minutes. Put the peppers in a small bowl and cover the bowl with plastic wrap. Let the peppers cool until you can handle them. The charred skin should separate from the flesh easily. (If not, let the peppers rest some more.) Cut off the stem, slice down the pepper, and scrape away the seeds, being careful not to touch them. (If you want the millet to have some real heat, save a few seeds. Be careful, though. They will surprise you.)

Preparing the millet. Set a teakettle full of water to boil. Meanwhile, heat a large pot over medium-high heat. Add the millet and stir continuously until it begins to pop. Some of the grains will turn a golden brown, and some may even look like tiny pieces of white popcorn. Do not let the grains burn. When the pot of millet smells toasted—about 7 minutes—pour in the boiling water from the teakettle. Add the butter and ¼ teaspoon of the salt. Simmer the millet over low heat until all the liquid has been absorbed and the millet is fluffy, about 15 minutes. Put the millet in the refrigerator until it has fully chilled.

Slicing the fruit. Peel and slice the mango and cut the fruit into bite-size pieces. Peel the jicama and cut it into matchstick-size pieces. Squeeze the juice from one of the limes over both the mango and jicama and place them in the refrigerator to marinate for at least 30 minutes.

Compiling the salad. Chop the roasted peppers and put them into the bowl of millet. Add the marinated mango and jicama. Peel the avocado and cut into small cubes. Add the avocado into the salad. Add the remaining ¾ teaspoon of salt, along with the cayenne pepper, and the juice of the remaining lime. Toss the entire mixture together. Marinate in the refrigerator for at least 2 hours.

Suggestions. This salad goes especially well with roasted chicken. You could also try topping the salad with a bit of soft goat cheese or thin slices of prosciutto.

Feeds 6.

quinoa

If you had asked me to point to the location of the Incan empire when I was in the fifth grade, I probably would have scrunched up my nose and guessed. Eventually, I would have admitted that I had no idea. If you had asked me the same question when I was in the eleventh grade, I would have done a better job of covering the fact that I still had no idea.

Education in my elementary school in the 1970s was fairly woeful. My teachers never knew what to do with me. Since I knew how to read at the age of two, my kindergarten teacher propped me up on a stool for story-reading time and had me read to all the other five-year-olds while she sneaked out of the classroom for a cup of coffee (and a cigarette, I suspect). In the fourth grade, my perpetually irritated teacher was further annoyed by the fact that I had set out to learn long division on my own time, and so she made me learn it again.

Global understanding certainly didn't rank high on my school's list of priorities. For my schoolmates and me, Latin American culture meant the annual pilgrimage in the yellow school buses to Olivera Street in Los Angeles on Cinco de Mayo. We kids stocked up on sweet Mexican candies and begged to burst the piñatas hanging above us on the street's tourist-trap stalls.

Geography education was even more inadequate, however. I don't ever remember being asked to look at a globe in a classroom or follow the trajectory of a river flowing to the sea. We were never asked to memorize state capitals or world cities. Honestly, I'm fairly sure we never looked at maps of any other country besides our own. The only reason I had a cursory knowledge of the layout of the United States was that I was once required to make a large-scale map of it, out of sugar cubes.

I do know how to sing all the states in alphabetical order, though. In choir, we learned how to sing "Fifty Nifty United States" for our cafeteria performances. If you asked me to sing it today, I could start chanting, immediately: "Alabama, Alaska, Arizona, Arkansas,

California, Colorado, Connecticut. . . ." Let me tell you, though, knowing the states in alphabetical order doesn't really help you navigate your way across the country on a road trip.

Thankfully, I know my geography better now. Becoming a teacher forced me to finally learn the capitals and the countries. (However, I still hope no one will ask me to sort out the states of the South.) Since I've gone gluten-free, I peruse maps the way I devour stories. Discovering quinoa taught me more about the Incas than my elementary school teachers ever did.

Quinoa is another in the line of unusual grains I've come to love since I found I needed to go gluten-free. The term "unusual" only means relatively unknown in the United States, because quinoa—like all these grains—has been grown for thousands of years across the world. The staple grain of the Incas, in Peru and Bolivia, quinoa is so densely packed with nutrition and protein that it allowed people to survive life at those high altitudes. For the people of the Andes, quinoa was considered one of the trinity of their most important foods, along with corn and potatoes. There are stories of the Inca emperor planting the first quinoa seeds of the season with a golden spade, in front of a gathered crowd. In that culture, for a time, quinoa seeds were more valuable than gold. Just as with amaranth, the growing of this gorgeous grain was abolished by the conquistadores in the seventeenth century. Some sources claim that this was because the Spaniards insisted that barley be grown instead, so they could make their familiar beer. And thus, over time, quinoa became illicitly grown, or grown only in remote places where people didn't have access to the bounties of the cities.

Quinoa was first brought into the United States in 1982, by the Quinoa Corporation. Representatives of the company bought a fifty-pound bag of quinoa seeds from Bolivia and tried growing it in this country. Again, as with amaranth, this was part of the natural foods movement to bring a series of grains into greater growing existence. Now quinoa is being grown throughout the United States, including my own western Washington state, since it needs cool summer nights for ideal growing. Commercially, it's available as a whole grain, as well as quinoa flour and pasta.

The raw grain has a coating called saponin, which is bitter. It's also so soapy that some scientists have suggested it should be used as a detergent. Most commercially available quinoa has the saponin already removed, but it's a good idea to rinse your quinoa before you start cooking with it. Also, when cooked in water or any kind of stock, quinoa swells to three times its original size, at which point tiny white bands appear across the middle of the grain. A friend of mine, upon first eating quinoa, exclaimed, "They look like worms."

Well, they kind of do. But they don't taste like worms. Quinoa is light to the taste and soft in the mouth.

Eating quinoa makes me feel better. According to the World Health Organization, quinoa is as high in protein as milk, with plenty of calcium as well. It's also filled with iron, B vitamins, zinc, and potassium. Apparently, NASA has played for years with the idea of sending quinoa with astronauts on long missions into space. Doesn't that make you want to try some?

Oh, and if you're wondering, it's pronounced KEEN-WA. You see, we learn something new every day.

When I lived in New York City, my best friend Sharon and I often went to brunch at a little French restaurant in the East Village called Danal. We'd descend the iron-railing steps to the door and then enter the cool cave of Provençal cuisine. Should we sit on the little patio or at the scarred wooden tables by the window? We'd order steaming bowls of café au lait as we looked at the menu. I don't know why we even looked at the menu, because in spite of our best intentions we always ordered the same meal, both of us. Little dill pancakes—the size of half dollars—with slivers of smoked salmon, a teaspoon of caviar, and dollops of crème fraîche. Every time, we'd close our eyes and exclaim at how good it tasted.

When I was first diagnosed with celiac disease, I didn't miss the idea of gluten much. After all, I had been so sick. But the thought of going to New York City and not ordering those little dill pancakes at Danal with Sharon made me genuinely sad. So I started making this quinoa and smoked salmon salad, with crème fraîche and fresh horseradish.

I don't miss the dill pancakes anymore, but I do miss Danal and Sharon.

Quinoa Salad with Horseradish Crème Fraîche

For the horseradish sauce

> ½ cup crème fraîche (or goat's milk yogurt)
> 2 tablespoons fresh grated horseradish
> ½ teaspoon kosher salt
> ½ teaspoon cracked black pepper

For the quinoa

> ¼ yellow onion, minced fine
> 2 cloves garlic, smashed and minced
> 1 tablespoon high-quality olive oil
> 1 cup quinoa, rinsed and dried
> 2½ cups chicken or vegetable stock
> 1 teaspoon kosher salt
> 2 roma tomatoes
> 1 orange pepper, cut into small strips
> 1 bunch green onions, chopped fine
> 1 head red leaf lettuce, rinsed, dried, and torn into bite-size pieces
> 4 ounces smoked salmon (optional)

For the vinaigrette

> ⅛ cup golden balsamic vinegar
> ⅛ cup balsamic vinegar (or ¼ cup, if you can't find golden balsamic)

1 teaspoon Dijon mustard
¼ cup high-quality extra-virgin olive oil
½ cup canola oil
salt and pepper to taste

Making the horseradish sauce. Combine the crème fraîche (or yogurt) with the grated horseradish, salt, and pepper in a bowl. Put the bowl in the refrigerator and allow the sauce to marinate for at least 30 minutes.

Cooking the quinoa. In a small skillet, sauté the onion and garlic in olive oil over medium-high heat until fragrant (about 2 minutes). Add the quinoa and toast it in the olive oil for about 1 minute. Add the stock and salt to the pan and bring mixture to a boil. Lower the heat to medium-low and let the quinoa simmer until it is tender (about 15 minutes). Spread the quinoa out on a plate and set it in the freezer for a few minutes to cool down.

Coring the tomatoes. Bring a pot of salted water to a boil. Take the cores from the two tomatoes. Flip them over and use a sharp knife to score a small x into the bottom of each tomato. Put them in the boiling water. When the skin starts to slip off, remove the tomatoes from the boiling water and submerge in a bath of ice water immediately. When they have cooled, peel the tomatoes, remove their seeds, and dice into small pieces.

Making the vinaigrette. Put the two vinegars, mustard, salt, and pepper in a blender and mix until well incorporated. Slowly, with the blender running, drizzle the oils into the blender until the vinaigrette has fully emulsified.

Assembling the salad. Take the quinoa out of the freezer (it should be well cooled but not at all frozen). Add the diced tomatoes, orange pepper, and green onions to the quinoa and stir. Drizzle a small amount of the vinaigrette over the quinoa and toss the salad. (Save the reserved vinaigrette for later salads.) Lay the quinoa on a bed of the red leaf lettuce. Top with the horseradish sauce and the smoked salmon, if desired.

Feeds 4, in small portions.

sorghum

In the 1990s, sorghum was ranked as the fifth most widely grown grain crop in the world, beaten only by wheat, rice, corn, and barley. How could there be a food that feeds millions of the earth's population, primarily in Africa and Asia, and I had never heard of it?

We have fallen into a food rut in this country. For decades—and particularly after the cult of convenience took over in the 1950s—we have stuck with wheat and more wheat, mostly stripped of its nutrition and made into white foods. Because of this tunnel vision and the myopic view that American culture is the only one worth investigating, we are missing the way much of the world eats.

Of course, I had never heard of celiac disease before I was diagnosed with it, either. We still have so much to learn.

Sorghum is a nutritious grain, originating in Africa, that is grown in voluminous quantities in the Midwest of the United States. In fact, sorghum was introduced into the United States in 1853, according to some sources. Today, the United States is the largest grower of sorghum in the world. However, here it is mostly grown as feed grain for cattle and poultry. Sometimes, it is even converted into wallboard and packing material. My friend Tita, who grew up in Wisconsin, knew about sorghum as a child, but she rarely ate it. There were rumors of popping the grain like popcorn, however.

One type of sorghum is called broomcorn, which is made into those rustic-looking brooms that seem to cost more at the store now than the artificial-substance brooms do. Another type, sweet sorghum, is made into syrups and sweeteners. Grain sorghum can be ground into a highly nutritious, wonderfully tasty flour. Indian grandmothers know how to make perfectly round rotis (or flatbreads) from sorghum flour, water, and salt by hand and heart. In Africa, sorghum is used to create porridges and to make beers, which heartens the hopes of those of us who must live gluten-free. In December 2006, Anheuser-Busch began mass-production of a gluten-free beer made of sorghum.

When I looked in my old hippie vegetarian books, I was surprised to find that not one of them mentioned sorghum. The index jumps straight from "snow peas" to "soups." It seems that sorghum flour was only recently made available on a large scale in the United States, and it's still mostly sold in specialty stores. I have experimented with sorghum flour in many recipes, and I have come to adore it. Its dense texture and slightly nutty taste gives it the heft of whole wheat without any of the gluten. Whenever I make gluten-free breads now, I always make the flour mixture at least half sorghum flour. It works wonders in flatbreads and scones as well.

However, I have found it almost impossible to obtain sorghum in its whole-grain state. I am certainly dedicated to pursuing good, gluten-free foods, but I have not been able to buy whole sorghum grains in Seattle. Maybe the growth of the gluten-free foods industry will heighten the awareness of sorghum and bring it to the masses. I hope so. Everyone should be eating this nutty, slightly sweet grain, not just those of us who have to go without gluten.

In the winter of 2006, the entire food blog world went seemingly insane for a no-knead bread recipe published in the *New York Times*. Oh, the raptures! Luisa at the Wednesday Chef made me want to try it, when she wrote, "Yes! A fantastic recipe! Something to rave about! Finally. What a relief." Looking at her bread, I knew I had to try it. Certainly, with all my skill and determination, I should have been able to make the bread by following the recipe and using gluten-free flours. Right?

In one word: no.

That recipe relies on the long strands of gluten that stretch and sway in the dough as it rises. Without gluten, what do you have? A blam-so-hard-you-could-break-a-tooth-with-it crust—good for defending against burglars—and crumbs so gummy that the bread tastes like no food in nature. It has more of a texture than a taste, and not a pleasant one at that.

Damn it. I wanted that bread.

However, after I wrote a funny post about the failure of the bread, I went back to it. I'm stubborn. I don't give up easily. My baking instincts told me that the key to the golden, crunchy crust on that bread was the Dutch oven and the 500-degree oven. After a week of varying the ingredients, I pulled a loaf out of the oven that made me gasp: light, airy, and with an incredible crust.

I still make one of these loaves of bread nearly every other day.

Crusty Sorghum Bread

2 teaspoons active dry yeast
1 teaspoon sugar
½ cup warm water
1½ cups sorghum flour
½ cup brown rice flour
½ cup sweet rice flour
½ cup tapioca flour
½ cup potato starch
2 tablespoons flaxseed meal
1 teaspoon xanthan gum
2 teaspoons baking soda
1 teaspoon salt
1 tablespoon apple cider vinegar
2 eggs
2 tablespoons high-quality extra-virgin olive oil
club soda at room temperature

Activating the yeast. Combine the yeast, sugar, and warm water. Mix gently in a large bowl and set aside until the mixture has combined and swelled to twice its original size, which should take about 15 minutes.

Preheating. Preheat the oven to 200 degrees F.

Combining the dry ingredients. Put the sorghum flour, brown rice flour, sweet rice flour, tapioca flour, potato starch, flaxseed meal, xanthan gum, baking soda, and salt into the bowl of your stand mixer. Turn on the mixer and combine the flours and other dry ingredients well.

Adding the liquids. Add the yeast mixture into the dry ingredients. Mix until just combined. Add the apple cider vinegar, then the eggs, one at a time, and then the olive oil. Allow the mixer to beat them into the dry ingredients, on low speed. Pour in the club soda in a slow drizzle. Pour in only as much as is needed to wet all the ingredients completely. The dough should feel soft and firm, like a baby's bottom.

Kneading the dough. Attach the dough hook to the mixer and stir the dough on medium speed for 5 minutes. This will give the dough a chance to cohere more evenly. It will also whip air into the dough, which will cut the usual density of gluten-free bread. After 5 minutes, turn off the mixer and transfer the dough to an oiled bowl. (If you do not have a stand mixer, knead the bread by hand on a gluten-free-floured surface, for at least 10 minutes.)

Allowing the dough to rise. Turn off the oven. Put the bowl into the oven, with a damp towel over the top of it. Leave the bowl in the oven for 90 minutes. The dough will not have risen much, at this point. There is no gluten to stimulate that rising. Accept that.

Baking the bread. After 1 hour, take the bowl out of the oven and put it on the stovetop to continue rising. Turn the oven on to 500 degrees F. Put a cast-iron pot, large enough to hold the bread, into the oven. (A cast-iron Dutch oven with an enamel surface is ideal, but any large pot or pan will do, as long as it has a lid.) Leave the Dutch oven in the oven for 30 minutes. Meanwhile, the dough will continue to rise on the stove.

After 30 minutes, carefully take the Dutch oven out of the oven. Without worrying too much about a perfect shape, transfer the wet dough into the hot Dutch oven. Put the lid on and immediately push the Dutch oven back into the hot oven.

Do not turn down the heat. Allow the bread to cook for the entire 30 minutes. By the end, it will smell like freshly baked bread. Take the Dutch oven out of the oven, remove the lid, and voilà—a wonderfully crusted loaf of gluten-free bread. Allow the bread to cool for 10 minutes, then cut right into it.

Suggestions. For olive bread, add ½ cup of chopped kalamata olives into the dough. For rosemary bread, add 1 tablespoon of chopped fresh rosemary into the dough, then sprinkle thick crystals of sea salt on the top of the bread before baking. Be creative. At the end of the evening, slice up any remaining bread and put it into the freezer. Gluten-free bread usually turns rock hard the next day.

Feeds 6.

teff

Summer 1985. I'm eighteen years old, about to turn nineteen. I'm sitting on the shag carpeting of my living room, in front of the television set, sipping a diet soda. My best friend, Sharon, is sitting there with me. We're snacking on rice cakes, out of guilt, although the potato chips, the sandwich cookies, and the pizza—straight from the freezer to the oven—will emerge several hours later. We're sitting as some small attempt to do our part for the cause. You see, we're spending that hot, Southern Californian summer day watching Live Aid, the international rock star telethon for the famine in Ethiopia. The images of starving children with flies about their faces, interspersed with performances by Sting and U2, was all I knew about Ethiopia at the time.

For the next fifteen years, that's all I ever knew about Ethiopia: a vague image of sadness and starvation. When I was a kid, I had never even heard of foods from Africa, much less Ethiopia. When I was in my twenties, I heard someone talking about visiting an Ethiopian restaurant, and I giggled behind my hands when someone else made a joke about what was served there: nothing!

I'm so embarrassed now. I had no idea what I was missing. Warm, spiced meals made with fenugreek and lamb. Soft, airy bread and tangy yellow cabbage, cooked until it's soft. Communal eating that clears the senses.

I introduced a good friend to his first Ethiopian meal at a tiny cáfe in Seattle, which looks ramshackle and even boarded up from the outside. In order to reach the six-table dining area, we had to walk through the small Ethiopian grocery store. All the spices needed to make my own veggie combo at home were contained on their sloping metal shelves. Everything was enshrouded in clouds of incense smoke. Inside the cafe, the windows were steamed up from the cooking. They didn't even offer menus. We had to know what we wanted.

There are no forks involved. Instead, we tore portions of the injera bread—spongy and slightly sour, with the consistency of a yoga mat—and pushed it into the cooked yellow cabbage and spicy lamb. All formalities disappeared. We talked and laughed as we bumped fingers over the Ethiopian cheese or chicken wat or beef kitfo.

Pete couldn't believe the taste. "It's fantastic. It doesn't taste like anything else I've ever eaten." He's right. It's much better than packaged cookies and frozen pizza.

The entire meal, for both of us, cost ten dollars.

In case you have never eaten Ethiopian food—and you must rectify that soon, if it's true—you should know that various spiced lentils, vegetables, and meat arrive arrayed on a large platter of injera bread, which is made from teff flour.

(Gluten-free readers beware: at some Ethiopian restaurants geared toward typical Americans, they might mix the teff with wheat or barley flour. Be sure to ask.)

Teff (also spelled tef or t'ef) is the staple grain of Ethiopia. This gluten-free grain is packed with protein, calcium, and iron. In fact, one cup of cooked teff contains as much iron as the U.S. Department of Agriculture recommends for adults in one day. It's nutritionally rich because most of the grain is made up of bran and germ, where the nutrients live. The whole grain is made into flour. The name, in Amharic, means "lost," perhaps because each individual grain of teff is so small—150 teff grains equals the weight of a single wheat grain—that it would be lost if dropped.

Teff was almost lost to the world. Grown exclusively in Ethiopia for thousands of years, teff was cultivated by Coptic Christians there. Isolated by their geography and religion from the rest of Africa, the teff farmers did not trade their grain, which is also labor intensive to grow. After Haile Selassie was deposed in 1974, the socialist military government of Ethiopia insisted that the farmers grow less labor-intensive crops, such as wheat, to export to other countries and to make more money for the state. Teff farming was beginning to die out. An American from Idaho, Wayne Carlson, was working as an aid worker in Ethiopia in the 1970s. Fascinated by the growing practices he witnessed, and having fallen in love with Ethiopian food, he took some of the teff seeds back home with him when he left. From there, he started growing teff in Caldwell, Idaho, then selling it to the Ethiopian communities in U.S. cities. Today, every bit of teff eaten in the United States comes from those seeds Wayne Carlson brought back from Ethiopia.

Thank goodness for the strange set of circumstances that allowed me to buy teff in a little ramshackle grocery store in Seattle. Since going gluten-free, I have come to adore teff.

Nutty in flavor and fine in texture, teff feels essential to gluten-free baking. Baked goods made with some portion of teff are soft in the mouth, melting almost immediately. Teff flour makes an excellent pie crust when you cut it with another gluten-free flour, such as rice flour or millet. In fact, it might be the best pie crust you've ever tasted. Teff flour, being so soft, and slightly gelatinous when it cooks, makes a perfect ingredient for baking quick breads. I'm certain that once you try it, you'll be as reliant on teff as I am.

Not cooking with teff? That's so 1985.

My mother came from a Pennsylvania Dutch background, so she could bake a pie better than anyone else I have ever met. Our freezer may have been stuffed with boxes of frozen pizza and spinach, but I never found a premade pie shell in there. The woman could bake.

I'm happy that she passed some of that on to me.

Baked goods served by the same hands that made them taste infinitely better than anything a manufacturer can produce. Moreover, baking from scratch is wonderfully inexpensive in comparison to buying a box. Making banana bread is especially thrifty, because bananas going soft really cannot be used for anything else. There is nothing like home-baked banana bread for a morning repast. This chocolate banana bread is the best of my grandmother's and mother's worlds: thrifty and decadent both. With the gluten-free flours—rice flour and teff flour, predominantly—it is mine. When I sit down and serve this bread to my friends for breakfast, there are only sighs of pleasure.

Chocolate Banana Bread

3 large bananas, mashed
½ cup butter, softened
½ cup organic cane sugar
½ cup turbinado sugar
2 eggs
1 teaspoon vanilla extract
½ cup sour cream
1 cup teff flour
½ cup sweet white rice flour
½ cup sorghum (or brown rice flour)
½ cup tapioca flour
½ cup almond meal (or hazelnut flour)
1 teaspoon cinnamon
1 teaspoon salt
1 teaspoon xanthan gum
1 teaspoon baking powder
1 teaspoon baking soda
3 tablespoons cocoa powder
3 tablespoons demerara sugar

Preparing for baking. Preheat the oven to 350 degrees F. Butter a 9-inch round cake pan. Flour the dish with a sprinkle of white rice flour.

Mashing the bananas. Mash the bananas with a large potato masher or a fork and set aside.

Creaming the butter and adding the liquids. Mix the butter and cane and turbinado sugars together. When they are just creamed, stop mixing. Add the eggs, vanilla extract, and sour cream to the butter and sugar. Mix in the mashed bananas.

Mixing the dry ingredients. Stir together all the dry ingredients. Break up the lumps of cocoa powder with a fork. Set aside.

Combining everything. Using a rubber spatula, fold the dry ingredients into the wet batter, ¼ cup at a time, until everything is just mixed together.

Baking the bread. Scrape the dough into your pan. Top with the demerara sugar, covering the surface of the dough. Place into the oven and bake for about 40 minutes, or until a knife inserted gently into the center of the bread comes out clean.

Cooling and serving. Let the bread sit in the pan for 5 to 10 minutes, then turn it over onto a wire rack. Serve warm, with cream cheese, if you wish.

Feeds 6.

There is, of course, so much more to know about these grains. I could go on for pages about the tastes and histories of each one. There are other possibilities for baking as well, including mesquite flour, chestnut flour, tapioca starch, potato starch, and cornstarch. I am still exploring, of course. But rather than making this chapter into an exhaustive history and description of each of the gluten-free grains, I want to entice you to try them. This is probably sacrilege for a high school teacher—one who has spent nearly a third of her life assigning nightly reading homework to teenagers—but I have to say it anyway. There's only so much that book learning can do.

Experience is the greatest teacher. Buy some amaranth, millet, quinoa, and teff. See what happens when you eat them.

7

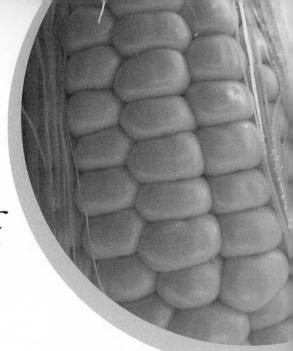

the pleasure of vegetables

I remember sitting at a long table, in a little plastic chair, waiting. In front of me sat a glass bowl of butter, already cooling.
It looked a touch disgusting but tempting, too. I waited with the
rest of my class for Mrs. Zee to bring us the next step. She placed
before me a plate of cooked leaves—gray-green leaves, steam rising
off them. Each leaf looked a little like a spiny cactus: daunting but
alluring.

I had never eaten an artichoke before. I had never even seen an
artichoke before.

After she had gone around the classroom and silently placed little
saucers of artichoke leaves before us, our soft-spoken teacher urged
us all to pick up a leaf. My fingers grabbed one and dropped it.
It was damp, a little spongy. The prickles tickled my hand. "Ew,
gross," I heard some other kids say. I thought so, too, but I hesitated
before I said it. I was fascinated. How could this be a food? In that
moment, I started to realize just how much I did not know.

Mrs. Zee quieted the cries, saying, "Try it. Even if you don't like
it, you'll have tried it." And so I dipped a damp piece of artichoke
in the glass bowl of melted butter and put it in my mouth. At first,

I only tasted the butter, salty and greasy. I liked butter, and I never had it often enough—we mostly ate margarine in my house—so I was willing to keep going. She told us to bite down, then drag our teeth up the leaf. It felt surprisingly thick, a little crunch along the edges, with a startling taste: like early mornings after a long, hard rain. I can still remember the sensory pleasure of scraping the flesh off that leaf with my teeth, the pleasure of tasting something I had never tasted before.

I kept dipping, more and more leaves, until I had eaten them all. Other kids in the class quit after one leaf. Some complained that this was just too gross. A few of us kept going.

I haven't stopped yet.

I don't know what possessed a second-grade teacher in Southern California in the 1970s to prepare fresh artichoke leaves for the seven-year-olds in her class. But I'm glad she did. The potency of the taste, the drag with my teeth, the ineffable pleasure of artichoke in butter—it is enough to fill an entire year of my life.

Compared with that glorious artichoke in second grade, eating vegetables in my house was rarely such a treat. Vegetables came from cans and frozen boxes, sometimes slathered in cheese sauce. I dreaded the days my mother pulled floppy bags of succotash from the freezer—nothing was worse in my child mind than cubed carrots, corn kernels, and vile little lima beans, all of them with that freezer-burn taste. If Mom insisted we eat our vegetables, she cooked the canned beans for ten minutes, and then coated them with margarine and salt. We ate potatoes as french fries, direct from the plastic freezer bag to the oven, crispy with oil and slightly burnt at the edges. Peppers arrived stuffed with ground beef, fried with a seasoning packet for flavor.

Other than the iceberg lettuce salads I ate nearly every night, I don't think I ever ate a vegetable on its own—in its raw, pure state—until I was in my twenties. Growing up, I never ate any eggplant, fava beans, or leeks. I did not know they existed.

I did love spinach, however. I craved the dark green taste of spinach, even though I had to open cans or packages to reach it. When I was a teenager, I came home from school, pulled a package of frozen spinach out of the freezer, ripped it open as fast as I could, threw it in the microwave, waited for it to stop spinning, squeezed lemon juice on the dark green leaves, and sat satisfied, five minutes later. What kid does this? Perhaps my body longed for the leafy green nutrition and iron of spinach, since I was always depleted. Some part of me wanted to live close to the earth, long before I knew the benefits.

It's strange. I grew up in Southern California, where fertile valleys yielding beautiful produce lie just outside the city. However, in the 1970s, that produce rarely reached our supermarkets. People simply did not have the expanded sense of the world's food we are starting to have now. Certainly no grocery store's produce section stocked romanesco broccoli—the lime-green, space-age curlicue of a vegetable related to traditional broccoli. We had broccoli.

When I was in my late twenties, I learned to eat raw vegetables. I was living on an island off Seattle, where earnest residents gathered in the small town square on Saturdays to sell their clutches of dahlias and hand-picked greens. This produce looked nothing like the vegetables I bought in the stores. It was pockmarked with holes at times, from worms and little bugs. It was smaller than the robust carrots that always came in uniform size, lined up in attractive bins and watered every seven minutes. These carrots were imperfect and strangely compelling. Every time I bought a new vegetable, I was amazed when I took it home and cooked it. My goodness—real taste.

I came to eat more vegetables because I had become a vegetarian. But the fact was that for me, vegetarian meant "not-meat," instead of an embracing of the leafy greens and bright colors that could have been decorating my plate. Sure, I ate my vegetables—and they were much better for being grown locally and organically—but I ate all the standard ones. I ate carrots with nearly every meal, excluding breakfast. I ate potatoes, tomatoes, broccoli, and green beans raw or cooked lightly. The day I bought snow peas to sliver into my stir-fry with brown rice, I felt adventurous.

Being forced to go gluten-free is what helped me to learn to love my vegetables. After months of exhaustion and pain—and especially after being reduced to eating jars of baby food to get nutrients into my system—I felt malnourished. This is no surprise to me now. After researching my digestive disorder, I learned that people who have celiac disease and eat gluten are damaging their small intestines. That's because the body reads gluten as a toxin, and it sends out antibodies to attack the offending food. In the process of going after the gluten, the antibodies attack the villi of the small intestines. These little fingerlike structures wave and ripple in the intestines, stretching out to grab food particles as they rush by. This is how our bodies absorb nutrition. However, in their attempt to attack gluten, the body's antibodies destroy major portions of the villi over time. This means that the body of someone who has celiac disease attacks itself and cannot absorb nutrition. Someone with active celiac sprue is malnourished, even if she is eating more than a jar of baby food at a time.

After going gluten-free, the first food I ate was a small plate of sautéed spinach. That leafy green had never tasted so good. After three weeks of eating gluten-free, I experienced sudden spasms of energy so enormous that I felt as though I could fly to the mountains on the power of my body. After months of feeling near death, I found myself dancing around the living room to songs I had forgotten I owned. I walked around the neighborhood so fast that I broke a sweat for the first time in months. I felt *good*.

Why? Because, after a lifetime of being malnourished and anemic, my body was finally absorbing nutrition properly. I was eating well and feeling the effects of it. I owed most of that to vegetables. Finally, I was able to let go of the past—frozen, flash-fried, and flabby—and learn to love my vegetables.

Of course, it's not just those of us who are forced to go gluten-free who should learn to love our vegetables. When I was reaching for a plastic bag in the produce section at my local market recently, I was struck by an absurdity. Printed on the bag, in big green letters, was "5 a day!" The store was cheerfully exhorting customers to eat at least five servings of fruits and vegetables a day.

Do people really need to be reminded of this? I guess we Americans do. I remember an isolated moment from the *Oprah* show sometime last year. I don't remember what the topic was, because I can only remember this moment: a woman in the audience admitted that she ate mostly fast food, all week long. The only vegetable she ever ate was the potatoes in the french fries. And she wondered why she suffered such bad constipation? I stared at the television set in cringing embarrassment for our entire culture. What are we doing to ourselves? Later that day, a friend of mine told me about her Thanksgiving weekend and said, "In four days of eating, there wasn't one green." I'm sure hers wasn't an isolated case. How did we become like this?

Why do we need to be cajoled to eat our vegetables, when they can be so damned good?

That same weekend, when my friend Monica came over on Saturday afternoon, I set a mushroom sauté in front of her made with chanterelles, creminis, and a pinch of Italian parsley, cradled in a touch of olive oil. She could not stop talking about the depth of taste in such a simple dish. I flash-sautéed green beans with almond slivers and sea salt. We ate fresh spinach salads with pomegranate seeds. Later in the evening, I slivered carrots thin and dusted them with cumin and honey before bathing them with olive oil in an extra-hot pan. Everything tasted fresh and redolent of health.

I can't imagine there is anyone reading this who does not know about the health benefits of vegetables. "Eating a diet rich in vegetables" is a phrase so ubiquitous in magazine articles about healthy eating that we should be able to recite it from memory. A diet rich in vegetables is said to prevent heart disease, strokes, various cancers, and high blood pressure. Eating the requisite number of vegetables every day can lower your cholesterol, give you healthy skin, and prevent type-2 diabetes. Eating vegetables high in dietary fiber helps bowel function, and we could all use that. Leafy greens, roots and tubers, cucurbita, caspiscum, pods and stems—they are all good for us. Eat a plethora of vegetables in every color across the spectrum, and you are bound to have a better life.

Really, who could have a problem with vegetables?

Well, I did, when I was a kid. I think that's where most of us have stayed: stubbornly in place. Learning to love vegetables takes an open mind and a willingness to change.

Thank goodness we have undergone a food revolution in this country. When I was a kid, I never ate shallots, mâche, fennel, or shiitake mushrooms. Now I consider them essentials in my pantry, staples of the season in which they grow. Even the biggest grocery stores now have three times as many vegetables in their produce section as the ones my parents shopped in when I was a kid. This is fabulous. It means we can all move beyond frozen spinach and canned green beans.

The summer after I stopped eating gluten, I started receiving a big box of organic produce on my doorstep every other Tuesday morning. A local produce company delivered organic, usually local, and just-in-season produce, all year long. Most cities in the United States now have a similar service. With a bit of research, we can all find a local community-supported agriculture (CSA). With this program, small farms take subscriptions from local residents, who receive a weekly box full of fresh produce, free-range eggs, milk, or whatever else may be grown on that farm. By buying into this program, we help to support small farms and to create a relationship with the people who grow our food.

One of my favorite hours of the week is late Saturday morning, when I take a slow spin around my local farmers' market. Washington state is blessed with good weather and fertile land, so there is much to choose from here. But it's not just the fat heirloom tomatoes or crinkly leaves of black kale that keep me coming back to this parking lot that is transformed into a village square every Saturday. It's the connection with the people who grow my food. There is the man from Olsen Family Farms, the one with a long beard and dirt under his fingernails, who smiles when he sees me, then tells me about his kids, as I pick out a pound of his purple potatoes. There are the immigrants who own Mai Cha Gardens and sell the most aromatic herbs I have ever smelled. The woman at the Whistling Train Farms always has the sweetest shy smile, as she points me toward her dandelion greens or daikon. Sometimes her daughter plays in the area behind her, crunching on baby carrots. In the corner of the parking lot sits a massive white tent, under which live every kind of pepper and chile imaginable. When I buy a pound, I give my money to a ninety-year-old man. He may be a little slow with the change, but he has been growing this food for the majority of his life. The women at Willie Green's laugh and tease one another, then grow serious as they tell their customers about their organic salad greens.

Finally, I always make a stop at Foraged and Found Edibles, run by Jeremy and Christina. For the most part, they make their living by digging in the rich earth of the woods in the Pacific Northwest and finding the best mushrooms growing at the moment. (When mushrooms are not growing, they take catering jobs.) They sell chanterelles and lobsters, oysters and morels, whatever is yielding itself to their hands that week. Then they make their rounds of the best restaurants in the city, walking in during the afternoon, before dinner service, and handing over mushrooms only hours away from the forest to the chefs, ready in their kitchens. I pick up a pound of porcinis, even though they are expensive, because I know they will feed me all week long, no matter how I cook them. I wave good-bye to Jeremy and head back to my car, loaded down with bags of fresh vegetables, and brimming with ideas of what to cook in the coming days.

Going gluten-free has guided me to think about how to eat locally, choose organic, and experience every taste I take more vividly. It has been a gift.

After living through an entire season cycle of eating gluten-free, I learned one lesson most profoundly: pay attention to the rhythms of the seasons. Since every vegetable I ate as a kid came packaged and frozen, I honestly didn't know that vegetables had seasons. I just assumed I could eat my microwave spinach any day of the year. Wasn't it always growing? But now I know more. Now I eat vegetables only when the earth wants me to eat them. And in doing this, I'm also paying more attention to what my body wants.

In summer, when the light stays late, and everyone feels light in the chest, I have boundless energy to cook and to create. Everything feels fresh and emerging. I eat vegetables straight from the stand. In autumn, however, everything grows a little darker. I start to slow down. In winter, we go into hibernation mode. The foods should correspond. If I eat in season, and plan meals in my kitchen according to the ingredients the earth is offering, then I feel better. Besides that, what would be the joy of baby artichokes in season if I could eat them all year long?

In the first year after I found out I had celiac disease, I tried more vegetables than I knew existed. Once I understood how malnourished my body had been for years, I made myself a pledge: one new vegetable a month. I decided either to try a vegetable I had never eaten or to dive back into the taste of something I had rarely eaten in its natural state. I was always enlivened. I consider it quite the coup that I finally took a bite of cauliflower and liked it. There are, of course, three dozen kinds of vegetables I cannot cover in this chapter, and a thousand variations on the ones I am featuring here. The snap of carrots, the crunch of red peppers, the bite of chard—the textures alone are enough to send me into ecstasies. But these are the vegetables I first learned to eat, or more deeply appreciate, because I started living my life gluten-free.

fennel with françoise

Three weeks after discovering that I had celiac disease, I went to a friend's house for dinner. This would be the first meal prepared by someone else's hands since I had stopped eating gluten. Potentially, I could have been nervous.

However, this invitation came from Françoise and her family. I hadn't been over in months, due to my illness, and I had missed their joy. Françoise is one of my favorite people in the world, *absolument*. Always, she smiles. Everything helps her discover something tremendous about life. She acts on that knowledge—so much of life is tremendous. And so I went to Françoise's for dinner, for "our first gluten-free meal!" as she put it. Camille and Selene danced around the kitchen in their stocking feet. Adriaan barbecued us salmon and bacon-wrapped scallops on the porch, even though it was pounding gray rain, unexpectedly. "Seattle barbecuing season," as he said.

One more check on the haricots verts in the pressure cooker, and then it was time for dinner. We sat down, with orange juice and enormous smiles. Succulent slices of barbecued salmon. Scallops with smoky bacon. Crisp green beans with almonds. A salad with wild greens and fresh dill from the garden, with a shallot and Dijon mustard vinaigrette. And a simple lemon fennel.

Fennel—I had never eaten it before. Françoise sliced it into thick slivers and dressed it in olive oil, lemon juice, salt, and pepper. I took my first bite, and I could hardly believe the beauty of it. Crisp and green, evocative of spring—it had a faint taste of licorice. I wanted as much of it as I could eat. The plate was full for only a brief time. The girls and I dipped our fingers into the plate, repeatedly. That sliced fennel was more addictive than french fries.

Life is full of small sweetnesses. Leave the brain fog and stupor of gluten behind, and everything looks beautiful.

Shaved Fennel with Lemon Juice

2 large fennel bulbs
⅓ cup high-quality extra-virgin olive oil
¼ cup fresh lemon juice
½ teaspoon sea salt
½ teaspoon cracked black pepper

Preparing the fennel. Remove the thick roots of the fennel bulb. Discard the leafy fronds and the thin white stems of the fennel. This should leave you with the thick, white portion of the fennel bulb. Shave the fennel with a mandoline, taking care to avoid cutting your fingers. If you do not have a mandoline, use your sharpest knife to cut the fennel bulb into slices about ½ inch thick. Let them fall loosely from the bulb and onto a plate.

Marinating the fennel. When you have finished slicing the fennel, mix the olive oil and lemon juice together in a small bowl with a whisk. Pour the liquid over the sliced fennel and toss it all together. Season with the salt and pepper.

Suggestions. If you let the dressed fennel stand for 10 or 15 minutes, the full flavor of the mixture will come out singing.

Feeds 5 (if 2 of them are ravenous children who like their vegetables).

picking baby carrots with a toddler

I am walking, with great care, through a garden in the rain. It is the Monday after the end of the school year, and I am tired. That push through final exams, grading, graduation, and the inevitable evaluations is hell on a teacher. After a year of rising early, I want to flop in bed and not rise until three. But here I am, just after eight in the morning, dressed and awake, away from my home. What could entice me out of my bed on the first day of summer?

Digging in the garden with Elliott.

Elliott, my dear nephew, is two and a half at this point, and he is relentlessly adorable. An early talker, he has a precocious way of being that makes me pay attention. His parents needed to be at work, and the little guy's regular babysitter couldn't make it that day. And so, I volunteered to spend my first day of the summer break with my favorite two-year-old.

He asked to go outside. Technically, this was summer, but we were just outside Seattle, so it was cool and rainy. We put on our shoes and I pulled the hood of his rain jacket onto his head. We walked out to the garden.

Elliott pulled on my hand, eager to show me something. Excited, he pointed at leafy green fronds poking up from the ground. "Look, Shauna! Cawwots." He sounded so much like Elmer Fudd in that moment that I laughed out loud. Immediately, his face formed into a frown. He thought I didn't believe him. So he bent down and reached out with his small fingers. Unfortunately, he didn't have quite the strength or agility to perform the feat, so I bent down in the rain and helped him.

I tugged and tugged, and then I pulled up a small carrot. Sweet and tender, almost unprotected in the cold air, this carrot looked entirely different from the ones I bought in the store. Elliott jumped up and down, lighting up his toddler sneakers with the red lights on the soles. "A cawwot, Shauna! Daddy said we could eat cawwots!" So I picked a dozen more, keeping a close watch not to pull up the ones that were no bigger than my thumb.

Summer had arrived.

Later in the week, when I had caught up on my sleep and strolled around the farmers' market, I spotted a bunch of baby carrots. Thinking of Elliott, I bought them, and then I took them home for little snacks. The next week, I found I had to eat them again. No longer were they obligatory, the food I ate when I was trying to watch my weight. Now, they were the sweetness of Elliott and the first day of summer.

I went home that second Saturday and made carrot soup, flavored with the fresh madras curry powder I had just discovered at my favorite spice market, just below Pike Place. With coconut milk and a touch of ginger, the soup tasted like some of my favorite Asian restaurants and an early-morning summer walk with my nephew at the same time.

Curried Carrot Soup

3 tablespoons high-quality olive oil
4 cloves garlic, smashed
6 large carrots, peeled, quartered, and small diced

1 medium white onion, peeled and small diced

2 stalks celery, cut lengthwise and small diced

1 stalk lemongrass (optional), root end removed, and stalk
　　smashed and chopped

½ apple, cored and small diced

1 tablespoon curry powder (this will taste even better if you find
　　fresh curry spices and grind them yourself)

¼ cup sweet white wine, such as Riesling

1 can (12 ounces) coconut milk

1 piece ginger, about 1 inch in length, peeled and chopped

1 cup heavy cream

2 teaspoons kosher salt

2 teaspoons cracked black pepper

juice of 1 lemon, strained of pulp and seeds

1 teaspoon sugar

2 tablespoons unsalted butter

Sautéing the vegetables. In a stockpot, heat 3 tablespoons of olive oil over high heat, then add the garlic. Cook for 1 minute, stirring constantly so that the garlic does not burn. Add the diced carrots, onion, celery, and lemongrass. Turn the heat down to medium. Cook the vegetables, stirring as you go, for 5 to 6 minutes, or until they have softened.

Adding the flavors. Add the apple and cook for 1 minute. Add the curry powder and cook for 2 to 3 minutes, stirring to ensure the curry powder does not burn. Deglaze the pot with the wine.

Bringing in the liquids. Simmer for 7 minutes. Pour the coconut milk in the stockpot, then add enough cold water to cover the vegetables by 2 inches. Simmer on low heat for 15 minutes. Remove the pot from the heat and add the chopped ginger.

Pureeing the soup and finishing it. Puree the soup in a blender and strain it through a fine-mesh sieve. Pour the soup back into the pot. Add the cream. Bring the soup to a boil. Season with salt, pepper, lemon juice, and sugar. Whisk in the butter.

Serve immediately.

Feeds 6 to 8 people.

tomatoes at the
peak of season

The first week of August is a summer tease. Even though the weather is hot and dry, with the sun high in the sky until late, the first fringes of autumn are in the air. The sun sets at eight instead of ten. There is a tiny tinge of chill in the evenings, presaging the coming months of cold. And in my mind, I start the inevitable countdown to the first days of school, alarmingly too soon. I want summer to last forever. I know that it won't.

My best consolation for this approaching end of summer is to walk into Sosio's and spot them: heirloom tomatoes. Fat and red, lumpy and orange, puckered at the edges and wonderfully imperfect, these tomatoes have a taste like no other. They taste like all the condensed sunlight of July, offered up to me in August.

Before I went gluten-free, I did not pay attention to my food the way I do now. In fact, I often bought pale tomatoes in January, their fat pink globes taunting me in the taste. Now I eat only fresh tomatoes during this time of year. I miss them in January, when I dream of that plump red goodness. But when they return, I devour them until I am sated, happy for the chance to eat something when the earth wants it to be eaten.

When it is tomato season, I make oven-roasted tomatoes, fresh tomato sauce for gluten-free pasta, and caprese salads with fat slices of tomato, fresh mozzarella, and basil leaves. I relish the chance to eat them for six weeks straight. Then I let them go.

Tomato, Fava Bean, and Gruyère Salad

1 pound fresh fava beans
1 tablespoon white balsamic vinegar
½ teaspoon Maldon sea salt (or your favorite sea salt)
½ teaspoon cracked black pepper
3 tablespoons fruity olive oil
20 grape tomatoes
¼ pound Gruyère
¼ pound finest prosciutto, sliced into small slivers

Preparing the fava beans. Set a pot of water, with a pinch of salt, to boil. Put a bowl of ice water in the sink. As the water is coming to a boil, shuck the fava beans. How to do this? Snap and extract. There should be 3 or 4 beans per pod. (Be sure to feel the inside of the pod, which is as soft as dryer lint.) When the water has come to a boil, plop all the shucked fava beans into the pan and let them bob in the boiling water for 30 seconds. After that, immediately drain the beans and plunge them into ice water. After a moment, drain the beans and chill them in the refrigerator for a few moments.

Making the vinaigrette. Put the white balsamic vinegar, sea salt, and pepper into the blender. Mix well. Slowly add the olive oil until the vinaigrette is cohesive.

Finishing the salad. Slice the grape tomatoes in halves, lengthwise. Cut the Gruyère into small squares, about the same size as the fava beans. Toss the fava beans, tomatoes, and cheese with the vinaigrette, then thread in small slivers of the prosciutto.

Feeds 2.

learning to love cauliflower

When I began to extol the virtues of vegetables to friends and strangers, inevitably people asked me, "Are there any vegetables you don't like?" Well, yes, I'd say. There are. And I'd rattle them off, like scripture off the tongue, my trinity: cauliflower, beets, and lima beans.

This was, as far as I was concerned, sacrosanct. Why change now? There are plenty of vegetables for me to make.

That's what I love about this gluten-free diagnosis. Instead of closing down my life, it has opened me up so entirely that I have become a different person. With restrictions in food necessary for my health, why shut down on everything else? Why not try those vegetables I once considered horrid?

In the middle of September, I learned to love cauliflower. I no longer simply accept it or have a fair-to-middling liking for it. I love it. Cauliflower just coos to me now. I see it in the store and head toward it. I've changed.

That fated day in September, I was at home, on a Friday, at four, chopping parsley and consulting recipes. Friends were due at seven, and I had ambitious plans. For days, I had been fiddling with the menu, trying to find the right fit.

Daniel has been feeding me for years—exquisite vegan food, on the balcony of his house, overlooking the garden. I can always count on eyes-closed appreciation moments there. Lisa was in the middle of a kitchen remodeling, so she was in no mood to cook. I wanted to feed everyone, and I wanted it to be good.

For appetizers, I lay out a goat-cheese marinade, a spicy hummus, Greek olives, and a Cocoa Cardona goat cheese from Wisconsin.

We ate a *soupe au pistou*, a warm medley of vegetables and pesto, from a recipe that Françoise gave me. There were millet fritters with cilantro and the first butternut squash of the season. And there was the roasted cauliflower.

A few weeks before, I had dinner with a fellow food blogger, who was in Seattle for a visit. As we talked about food and writing and more food, Matt mentioned that he was thinking of making cauliflower roasted with cocoa powder for his sister's dinner. What? I had never heard of it, but my mind turned toward it. Matt told me that he had learned to dust cauliflower with cocoa powder at the Culinary Institute of America—standard stuff there.

Hesitant at the thought of chalky, rigid cauliflower, I still hadn't made an attempt at the exotic dish yet. But I had friends over, people who were willing to be guinea pigs. Daniel had once made me sautéed cauliflower that had tasted surprisingly alert. He had been urging me to conquer my fears ever since.

As we laughed and talked, the guests in the living room, me in my familiar place before the stove, I tossed cauliflower florets in Spanish olive oil, sea salt, and pepper. At the last moment, I decided to toss on some smoky Spanish paprika, dark red with a kick. And then, with a fine-mesh sieve, I sifted on some unsweetened cocoa powder. A little chocolate and chile—mole sauce flavors. I had no idea how it would work.

Twenty minutes later, Daniel was exclaiming, Mane was groaning, Lisa was shaking her head in excitement, and I was just grinning. Earthy, rich roasted, layers of taste—this roasted cauliflower was unforgettable. I knew then that I could never again say, "I do not like cauliflower."

Roasted Cauliflower with Smoked Paprika and Cocoa Powder

2 tablespoons kosher salt
juice of 1 lemon
1 head cauliflower
3 tablespoons high-quality olive oil
½ white or yellow onion, thinly sliced
4 teaspoons smoked paprika
1 teaspoon unsweetened cocoa powder
1 teaspoon sea salt
1 teaspoon cracked black pepper

Preheating. Preheat the oven to 425 degrees F.

Blanching the cauliflower. Bring a pot of 2 quarts of water plus the kosher salt and the juice of half the lemon to boil. Cut the florets off the stalk of the cauliflower. Put the cauliflower in the boiling water and cook for 5 minutes. Drain and pour the cauliflower into a bowl full of ice water. Let it rest there for 3 minutes, or until it is chilled. Remove the cauliflower and pat dry.

Cooking the cauliflower. Bring a skillet to heat on high, then add the olive oil. When the oil runs easily around the pan, add the thinly sliced onion. Cook and stir until translucent and soft, 2 to 3 minutes. Add the smoked paprika. Add the cauliflower to this mixture and coat them well. Cook for 3 minutes, stirring occasionally, until the cauliflower is coated and the fragrance of the paprika is strong. Remove the skillet from the heat.

Roasting the cauliflower. Add the cocoa powder to the cauliflower. Add the salt and pepper. Toss the cauliflower to coat. Transfer this mixture to a roasting pan. Put in the oven and cook the cauliflower for 5 minutes. Drizzle the remaining lemon juice over the cooked cauliflower.

Feeds 4.

asparagus—that vivid green of spring

Sometimes, the best pleasures are the simplest.

One balmy day, Merida and I took a long walk around my neighborhood, marveling at the warmth of the air along our arms, which were bare against the sun for the first time in months. Boys were bouncing basketballs against the sidewalk as they walked home. People's chests were opening outward, like buds unfurling into flowers. We heard someone running his lawn mower along the grass of his front yard, from blocks away. We both said, "It's spring."

Later, at my favorite produce stand, when I asked what was best that day, the man serving me simply pointed to the asparagus. Full as pregnant pauses, more lurid green than anything in nature the past four months, this asparagus looked splendid. It came from California, instead of my attempted one-hundred-mile radius. But these were the first harbingers of spring. More than that, it was the one-year anniversary of my celiac diagnosis. I had now been living gluten-free for a year, and I felt gloriously alive. Some people would have drunk champagne. Me? I bought myself some asparagus.

Throbbing with spring green taste and mellow sweetness, asparagus never fails to delight me. That authentic green taste comes rushing sweet as a first kiss at the end of the evening. Recipes don't have to be complicated to satisfy completely. This time of year, I roast asparagus in good olive oil and balsamic vinegar nearly every day. I nibble up the long spears, hot out of the oven, as an afternoon snack. If, somehow, I manage to restrain myself and save some for the next day, I slice them up for salads with slivers of parmesan cheese, or toss them in egg white scrambles with smoked salmon. Somehow, roasted asparagus is spring to me.

Roasted Asparagus

1 bunch fresh asparagus, of medium thickness
2 tablespoons high-quality olive oil
1 teaspoon sea salt
1 teaspoon cracked black pepper
1 teaspoon balsamic vinegar

Preparing. Preheat the oven to 450 degrees F. Fill a large pot with 1 to 2 inches of water. Bring to a boil. Set a large bowl full of ice water in the sink.

Blanching the asparagus. Cut off the thick, woody ends of the asparagus and rinse each of the spears. When the water comes to a full, roiling boil, put the asparagus spears in the water. Let them bob around for 1 to 2 minutes, depending on the thickness of the spears, until they turn a tender spring green. Using tongs, lift the asparagus spears out of the water.

Shocking the asparagus. Immediately, dunk the blanched asparagus spears into the ice water, which is known as shocking the asparagus. This will arrest the cooking process. After a moment, lift the asparagus spears from the ice water and dry them off.

Roasting the asparagus. Pour the olive oil into the bottom of a skillet. Toss the asparagus spears in and coat them with the oil. Season them with the salt and pepper. Put the skillet in the hot oven.

After 3 or 4 minutes, the asparagus spears should be sizzling audibly and become soft enough that a fork will go in easily. Don't overcook, or they will wither into themselves. Let them be a vivid spring green.

Serving the asparagus. Remove the asparagus spears from the oven. Drizzle them lightly with the balsamic vinegar. You want the depth and unexpected sweetness of it, but not the acrid tang of too much vinegar.

Feeds 2, if you want to share this with someone special.

8

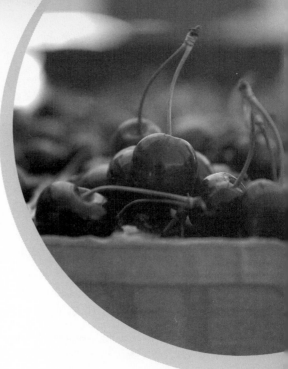

luscious and sumptuous fruit

In the backyard of the house where I spent the bulk of my childhood grew a pomegranate tree, crowded up against the cement
patio. It shadowed the small square of gray where I learned to roller-
skate on my large, clunky wheels. In the autumn, my bisected arc
was cut even shorter by the splat of murderous red etched onto the
gray cement. That tree grew so many pomegranates, overly large and
ready to split, that they fell to their deaths, cracked on the cement,
splayed open. The blue jays came by to steal their seeds. The patio
was smeared with sticky red until the torrential rains of December
came and washed it all away for another year.

This pomegranate tree, in the pounded-down dirt of a small
Southern California lawn, seemed normal to me. Early on, I
regarded the exotic as daily, necessary, something like home. However, I don't remember eating any of the pomegranates from that
tree. I only remember trying to skate around the red stains. It took
me twenty years to finally open a pomegranate. A fellow food blogger (Brett from In Praise of Sardines) taught his readers a trick for
how to remove the seeds without dealing with the pith. Split the
pomegranate in half, score the top of the pith lightly with a knife,

turn over the pomegranate, then smack the back of it with a solid wooden spoon. Remarkably easy, this trick works every time. (It is also helpful for channeling aggression.) I love seeing the red stain of pomegranate juice directly on my hands instead of skating around it on that old cement patio.

I never would have eaten the seeds directly from the fruit if I had not gone gluten-free. Desirous of as much nutrition as I could get after years of being malnourished, I sought out every fruit I could eat. When September sauntered into town, I remembered the vivid images of pomegranates splattered on the ground, and I wanted to eat them. (Maybe I also wanted to eat up those memories of childhood and digest them fully.) Pomegranate juice had made its debut on the market a year before as the latest health fad in food. Squat, curvy bottles of the rich crimson liquid started showing up in the refrigerated portion of the produce section, at nearly five dollars a bottle. Much as I loved that tart taste and tried to extend the life of the bottle by cutting the juice with water, that was just too much to pay for juice. I ate the fruit instead.

The fleshy seeds of the pomegranate, rich in red, juicy in the mouth, may have taken a few moments to extract, but that made them all the more worthwhile in my eyes. They looked like little magenta teeth. I adored their harsh sweetness, the crisp crunch of the little seeds that seem to not yield at first. They need concentrated chewing. After the first burst of overpowering taste, like little fists pounding at the inside of the mouth, the flavor drops away and they become mainly texture. Lingering. Singular.

After this, possibilities of pomegranates danced in my head. The seeds added sweet bite to homemade guacamole. Pomegranate molasses started slipping into meat dishes in the evenings. Squeezing the seeds through a fine-mesh sieve one day, I found out how to make my own juice, much cheaper than the one in bottles. I ate pomegranates all autumn long, while the fat globes were stacked up in piles at my local grocery store.

This is what has happened to me since I went gluten-free. Instead of searching for pale substitutes of what I used to eat, I sought out foods that I had never eaten before, simply because they do not contain gluten. To my surprise, I found that the foods intrigued me and then quickly felt indispensable to me. I began creating dishes with confidence and abandon, not consulting any recipe, just following my tastes. Eventually, I figured out how to make something from scratch that I had only bought in a store before. I felt triumphant, and I ate well.

Thank goodness for going gluten-free.

There is something luscious about fruit, something decadent and sensual, yielding and pliable, something essential. It's no wonder that Eve was seduced by an apple instead of a stalk of celery. Try to imagine life without the soft bite of a pear, the plump softness of a raspberry, the tart directness of a lemon, the mouth-puckering chew of a blackberry.

And yet, so many people don't eat fruit. Or they find it in their diets in horribly disguised fashions. Honestly, when I was a kid, I probably ate more Hostess fruit pies than raw pieces of fruit. At school, our lunches arrived with minuscule fruit cups, which swam in sticky syrup, topped with a lurid-red maraschino cherry. Powdered kid drinks left my upper lip stained with fruit-punch coloring from #2 dye, but I don't think there was actual fruit in any of them. Otter Pops may have come in fruity flavors, but were there any actual blueberries in the Louie Blue Blueberry frozen treat? Pizza parlors across the country added a Canadian bacon and pineapple pizza to their menu in the early 1980s, which may have given me a quarter cup more of my daily fruit requirement than I had been eating. I was capable of blowing prodigious bubbles with my Juicy Fruit gum, but I can't imagine that helped my nutritional intake. Hard candies came in raspberry and lime flavors, sugary cereals with fruit in the name bobbed at the top of my bowl of milk, and sometimes strawberry jam lay beneath the layers of white-flour crust and sticky frosting of that popular toaster treat.

When I was a kid, I ate each of those foods with as much avidity as my peers. We were a snacking generation, brought up to eat those vending-machine foods as though they were mother's milk. But now that I am an adult, I can only say, "Eeeeew!" When was the last time you actually touched the top of a packaged fruit pie? They are stiff and nubbly, with a texture created by the deep-fried sugar like nothing known to the natural world. I wouldn't eat one now if you paid me, even if I could eat gluten.

So much of packaged food feels and tastes like a simulacrum of real food, but especially the fruit-flavored foods that so many of us grew up eating. As with all packaged foods, fruit foods are overly sweet. When someone who has grown up on junk food first tastes a real raspberry instead of a raspberry-filled Danish, he may be startled by the taste. Instead of a flat, too-sweet gloppiness, a real raspberry has a soft cup of texture, little prickles on the skin, a hollow center, and a tartness only overtaken by a singing-out sweetness after the first bite. None of that shows up in fruit flavoring in food. It never will.

There is something primal in fruit. All great food, for me, has the ability to stop time. One bite, and I am no longer consumed with myself. Instead, I am merely someone chewing, someone experiencing that bite of food. Most fruit at its perfect ripeness has the feeling of soft, human flesh, a little plump with a lot of firm give. Think of a mango at the moment you need to eat it, or an apricot, or a plum. However, an autumn apple eaten ten minutes after it has been picked has a rich stiffness. Pay attention to the way your jaws almost seize up with the tartness, how your mouth releases saliva at the sweetness, how each bite has the crunch of walking in new snow. And there are the shreds of apple skin that stick in the teeth, clinging to the hope of being eaten. No glass of apple juice—even if it is 100 percent organic—can ever match the experience of eating an apple.

No question that everyone should eat more fruit, and not in processed foods and commercially baked goods. Fruit is rich in nutrients and dense in vitamins and can help prevent all kinds of diseases and minor maladies, if you eat it in the right quantity. When I first started eating gluten-free, the sun shone strongly for the first time after a long winter. I ate all the late-spring, early-summer fruits I could find, and I swore that I could feel myself growing stronger every day.

But some fruits might make you sick if you do not buy them organic. In the last decade, organic foods have begun appearing with increasing frequency across the country. In fact, sales of organic food have exploded by 20 percent over the past five years. Once the cause célèbre of fringe health food stores, organic produce, milk, meat, and eggs are now showing up in such mainstream places as Safeway. Of course, before the 1950s and the mass introduction of chemical pesticides onto the nation's produce, everyone ate organic. But never mind. Here we are, and we have to deal with how our food is grown right now. At the moment, there is no denying that organic food costs more than nonorganic food. Is it worth the extra price?

A few years ago, the Environmental Working Group researched thousands of pesticides and their effects on produce. After doing test after test on random samples of vegetables and fruit across the nation, the group revealed its Dirty Dozen list. These dozen are, in the estimation of the Environmental Working Group and other groups like it (including the U.S. Department of Agriculture), the fruits and vegetables that necessitate buying organic. Why? Because the nonorganic versions of these fruits and vegetables consistently tested high for pesticides, no matter where in the country they had been grown. So, if you want to avoid eating a big mouthful of chemicals with your fruit, buy organic apples, cherries, imported grapes, nectarines, peaches, pears, red raspberries, and strawberries. (For the record, the vegetables are bell peppers, celery, potatoes, and spinach.) It's fairly easy, really, to find farmers who grow organic, naturally, and buy from them directly. That organic strawberry at the height of summer won't feel so expensive as the one you find in stores, and it will taste much better than the conventional strawberry as well.

The summer I turned sixteen, I spent mornings in the pool, before it grew unbearably hot. In the afternoon, I stayed inside in shaded rooms, reading stacks of books, trying to avoid the scorching sun. The transition between the two halves of my day was lunch. Every day of that summer, I ate the same meal: an enormous egg salad sandwich, a tall glass of iced tea, and a mound of dark red bing cherries. There were a few memorable milestones that summer. In those long hot days, I discovered a keening, teenage-girl passion for the Beatles, after years of hearing them play in the background of my life. On those solitary afternoons, I spent hours with giant headphones on, listening to *Rubber Soul* as closely as I could. Those beautiful young men spoke to me, and I felt as though I was finally being heard. That summer is also when my agoraphobic mother began loosening her grip on my brother and me, just a bit. During that summer, I was allowed to ride my bike around the block by myself for the first time.

However, honestly, what I remember most clearly that summer was the taste of those cherries. After a childhood of eating very few raw fruits—aside from mushy Red Delicious apples—I felt my tongue exploding open when I ate those wine-dark fruits. With their sweet juice seeping out, firm flesh, and a generous chew, those cherries felt like being sixteen, crouched but ready to spring open. I ate the entire mound with a ritual-like intensity: plucking the stem from the cherry, splitting it open with my teeth, eating each half with my eyes closed to taste it more. And then I spat the pit into a waiting bowl, slowly filling it up with blood-rich pits. I ended every lunch with a satisfied sigh.

Early August, Vashon Island, somewhere in the early 1990s. My friend Julie and I are sitting on the beach. This is a Pacific Northwest beach, craggy rocks and slimy green algae drying in the sun, with water so cold that we start to howl if we stick our feet in it for longer than three minutes. Instead of surfing or sunbathing, we are sitting in the shade of evergreen trees, our toes stretched into the sun.

Julie has packed us a picnic, and we talk and watch her dog Scout frolic on the rocks, as she pulls everything out of the basket. Goat cheese and a crusty loaf of bread. A small salad with wild greens and a balsamic vinegar dressing. Slices of spicy salami. Squares of dark chocolate. Fizzy fruit juices to drink. What I remember best, however, came at the end of the meal. Julie, with tenderness, pulls out two peaches, fat and fuzzy, as gently pink at the edges as a young girl's blush. "This is peach season," she tells me. "This is the only time I eat them." These have come from east of the mountains. I can see from the glow around them that these peaches will be good. But I am not prepared. I take a generous bite, and peach juice dribbles down my chin. The high, clear sweetness of a perfectly ripe peach rings out to the water, followed by my exclamations. "How can a peach taste this good?" I ask her, almost sad at the memory of every peach I had eaten before. Then, I take another bite and close my eyes to experience this more fully. Summer sweetness, a tender flesh—the taste of indolent freedom. This is, finally, an object in the world that embodies succulence. I want to wallow in its juices and burrow into its flesh. I want to linger there for hours.

When I teach students how to write poetry, I cajole them to write with images instead of ideas. "Make me feel it with you. Capture the sensory experience in words," I tell them. And some of them understand, immediately. Others need examples. And so, I tell them that my first image of summer is the experience of eating that peach on a hot day on a beach on Vashon Island. The distillation of that experience is "the peach juice dribbled down my chin." After hearing that, they lower their pens to their papers and begin writing.

Early September. I am walking with my nephew, Elliott, in the wilds of the woods behind his house on Vashon Island. He swings his arms from side to side as he walks down the path, his sturdy little three-year-old body guiding him toward goodness. He leads me to a blackberry patch still yielding life, even though summer is nearly over. He puts up his hand, his fingers reaching for the fattest, blackest berry.

He plops it in his mouth, then chews down. Upon his face erupts a sweet smile like sunrise. I grab one as well, feeling the warmth of the sun on my fingers, the prickles of the berry trying to prevent me from eating it, and the juice already spilling from the purple pockets. Slowly, trying to enjoy the moment, I raise the berry toward my mouth. Aching beauty. Dark sweetness. A bit of tartness. The entire summer of freedom and loving and laughter and long nights concentrated into one taste. One glorious taste—blackberry.

Elliott turns toward me and says, "Blackberries are just my favorite, favorite fruit." And I agree.

Then he reaches for another one.

Eating ripe, organic fruit in season opens my senses to wonder. It is those moments of being open to wonder—in awe, aware, and glad to be alive—that I remember, decades later. If we eat good fruit, we create memorable bites for ourselves, bites that will stay with us all our lives.

Luscious persimmons, quixotic quinces, bulbous dragonfruits, dusty breadfruit, chubby cherimoyas, and enormous jackfruits—so many exotic fruits yet to discover. And yet, in season, there is nothing to equal the slithery sensuality of a ripe mango, the mild tartness of Meyer lemons, the burst of goodness of blueberries, the gasping relief of the first strawberry of spring. I will never grow tired of every attribute that fruit has to offer—honeyed, fragrant, mellifluous, or golden—and all the ways that I can eat it.

the joys of making jam

On a hot July day a few months after I found I had to go gluten-free, I made eleven jars of raspberry jam. Never having made jam before in my life, I decided to make it at ten at night, when the kitchen was cluttered with dishes to be done, and me in my favorite tank top that I didn't really want to stain. But I had bought a flat of organic raspberries at the farmers' market that day, and I suddenly realized I had to make jam *that night*.

My seventy-four-year-old friend Mary, who had been making jam for her family for nearly fifty years, talked me through how to make freezer jam as we bobbed in the pool that afternoon during a Hydro-fit class. I dried off and drove to Ballard, where they close off several streets to cars so that local farmers can sell their homegrown cheeses and wines, fit-to-burst peaches, and gorgeous Rainier cherries. A Jamaican man played the steel drums on the sidewalk in front of the peaches. Another man with shades played the electric guitar, contorting his face to emulate the blues. There was a moment in the middle of it all—a plastic bag stuffed with fresh fruit dragged on my left arm, and the sun shone through my smudged sunglasses—when I could feel my body open to all this happiness and just let go.

Somehow, I could taste all this in the jam later.

I had never made jam before, but after the gluten-free diagnosis, I no longer felt daunted. The more I cooked, the more I found something deeply satisfying about these domestic tasks. When I was younger, I had no time for these tasks, thinking them something that women in the 1950s did. But now I realize that cooking food, doing the dishes, and making jam are meditative acts. I planned on giving most of the jars away as gifts. I made jam as a way of loving people. And the jam tasted like raspberries, warmed in the sun.

I never would have made jam if I hadn't found out I had celiac disease.

Raspberry-Vanilla Jam

After I had been cooking for a while longer, I learned that making jam from scratch, without the pectin, is wonderfully easy. All it takes is patience and some stirring.

> 2 cups fresh-squeezed orange juice
> ½ vanilla bean
> 4 cups fresh raspberries
> ½ cup sugar

Boiling the orange juice. In a small saucepan, bring the orange juice and vanilla bean to a boil. Let the mixture boil for 15 minutes, until it has reduced a bit.

Simmering the berries. Add the berries and sugar to the orange juice mixture. Bring them to a boil, then lower the heat to a simmer. Let the berries simmer for 2 hours, stirring occasionally.

Finishing the jam. You will know when the jam is done when the berries have broken apart, the liquid has thickened, and it looks like jam. Spoon the jam into a small jar and refrigerate immediately. Use it within 30 days.

Makes a ½ pint of jam.

blackberries and salmon— this is seattle

I did a bad thing.

I bought blackberries.

Oh, there's nothing wrong with blackberries. In fact, there's everything right with them. Nothing can match the full-on explosion of sweet tartness, warm spikiness, and indelible pleasure on the tongue. Rolling waves of taste and memories jumbled into one. The summer sun on dust and black sugar kindness, and I'm waving hello to every berry as I pick it. I love blackberries.

No, the problem is—I bought them.

I'm so ashamed.

Here in Seattle, blackberries grow wild on the sides of the road in summer. Whenever I'm on my bike on the Burke-Gilman trail, my nose goes first. Fat cascades of blackberry bushes tumble down the hills around me, and I'm swathed in scented heaven. Seattle smells sweet in the summer. There are moments when I'm convinced I smell wild dill and basil among the blackberries. But somehow, I always forget to wear my backpack stuffed with plastic bags as I bike, so I can hop off and pick enough berries to makes pies and cobblers all summer. I just keep rolling, enjoying the smell.

When I lived on Vashon Island, nearly a decade before, every street yielded a fresh patch of blackberries. My friend Tita and I went picking all summer, filling old yogurt containers and little plastic buckets and jars full of the gorgeous black fruit. The juice ran down our fingers as we picked, and we ate, so that our nails were stained dark purple for days. Afterward, we'd walk back to her house, happy and sun-washed, talking away. We'd crowd into her small kitchen and immediately make a blackberry pie, then play Parcheesi with John, laughing into the evening. But that summer, Tita had mononucleosis and couldn't do much, so we couldn't make a pie in her kitchen.

Every summer since I moved to Seattle, I've been in Discovery Park, picking blackberries. Discovery Park has a plethora of bushes, just off the loop trail. Walk among old-growth forests, awed at the canopy of leaves above your head, then feel your body open wide as the trees fall behind, and you're looking at the expanse of Puget Sound. I've come out of every session with scratches on my arms and hands, as though a pack of feral cats were waiting in the bushes instead of blackberries. But the summer after my celiac diagnosis, I was so busy cooking and tasting and writing that I hadn't made it out to Discovery Park for blackberries. It felt too late.

I had to buy them.

I nearly didn't. There they were, offering up their burnished beauty in little green boxes at the West Seattle farmers' market. I passed by stall after stall, feeling too guilty to grab a box. But at one stall, I just couldn't resist the smell. Those berries seemed particularly juicy and plump. I told of my guilt, almost as a way to apologize. But the affable man selling them said the magic words: "Oh, you couldn't pick these by the side of the road. They're sweeter and have fewer seeds. And you know there are no pesticides or animal tracks on them."

Okay, I bought a pint. Or two. So sue me.

Besides, handpicked among thorns or bought with clean cash, blackberries please the mouth, enormously. When I turned those stall-purchased blackberries into a sweet, slightly spicy sauce to top sautéed salmon, it didn't really matter where I had found them. The sauce with a kick opened in my mouth with joy, just the way something with blackberries should.

Blackberry Sauce for Salmon

1 pint fresh blackberries (frozen will do, when they are out of
    season)
½ cup water
juice and zest of 1 lemon
2 teaspoons honey
½ teaspoon cayenne pepper
½ teaspoon balsamic vinegar

Cooking the sauce. Put all the ingredients into a small sauce-pan. Bring the mixture to a boil on medium heat. Lower the heat and simmer for 10 minutes, until the mixture has begun to thicken.

Pureeing the sauce. Puree the sauce in the blender. Strain it through a fine-mesh sieve. Taste the sauce to ensure it works for you.

Serving the sauce. Drizzle the hot sauce over pan-seared salmon.

Suggestions. This sauce also works well with roasted chicken or pan-seared pork chops. Try it on vanilla bean ice cream for an explosion of taste.

Feeds 4.

making pie in the big apple

Once, when I was living in New York City, I made an apple pie for a dinner party at my friend's apartment on 84th Street. Since I lived on 101st, I knew I wouldn't have far to go, and I was just too broke to take a cab for that little distance. So I decided to take the M104 bus. But planning ahead with food—the pie not only baked but also perfectly cooled before I climbed on a big-city bus with it—has never been one of my strong suits. I dashed around the kitchen, checking on the state of the fruit beginning to bubble softly in the slits of the top crust, and took time to dust the flour from my nose. One look at the clock told me I didn't have time to wait any longer. So I grabbed my purse, then I pulled the pie from the oven, and I went down the elevator with a hot apple pie in my oven-mitted hands.

Now granted, I'm sure this isn't a typical sight on the Upper West Side, but I had no idea what a commotion I would make. My doorman started first, craning his neck to see where that smell was coming from, down the hall. When he spotted me, he shouted, in his thick Albanian accent, "Hey! Can I have some?" I smiled genially and passed by. The guy outside, the one who always hung out at the stoop, grinned up at me as I passed, the only smile he ever gave me, and murmured, "Ah, pie. Now that's a woman." As I walked onto the street, I saw hungry eyes following me, fixed on the pie. When I entered the crosswalk, a trucker leaned down on his horn and startled me so much I nearly dropped the pie. He laughed and pointed at the pie. Shaking my head and laughing at the scene, I felt as if I were in a Fellini film about baking. I climbed onto the bus when it came. Fumbling with my MetroCard and trying to balance the pie on the card reader, I didn't look at the other people on the bus for a moment. But when I looked up, I saw that they were all staring at me. Every one of them. Even the guy in the back who usually sat slumped against the window, drooling. Every one of them was looking at me. No, they were looking at my pie. Suddenly shy, I ducked my head and walked down the center aisle, sometimes nodding at people as I went by. But I could tell that their stares followed me.

When I finally found an open seat, I scrunched down into it. The woman next to me fake-moaned, "Oh, you would have to sit next to me!" And then she said, "Can I have a piece?" To which I gamely smiled and half laughed, the way I was supposed to. But I've always wondered what would have happened if I said, "Okay!" then took out a knife and cut her a slice? (Another time.)

Just as everyone seemed to have settled down and grown used to the pie, we stopped at 96th Street. Something shifted in the air. An angry passenger climbed onto the bus. Full of frenetic energy, and furious at the world, the lithe man bent his body to bang on the card reader. Short of change, he grew furious at the driver, who finally let him just go to the back without paying. As he walked down the aisle, the man muttered to himself, and to us, about the state of the world—loudly, in vile language and with a hint of violence in the way he walked. Everyone froze. We all looked down at our laps, which left me looking at my steaming apple pie. I know the rule in New York: don't make eye contact with a crazy person. It will only make for trouble. I kept thinking, "Please don't take my pie."

But after a few more stops, I noticed that everything had become quiet. The air felt as if it was moving again. What had happened to the angry man? I looked up to see him by the back door, a smile across his face, his eyes suddenly delighted, all trace of violence gone. And he pointed at my lap, then laughed and said, "Pie!"

It seems that nothing brings New Yorkers together like a fresh-out-of-the-oven pie.

For a woman with pie stories, being told you can never eat gluten again is quite the shock.

However, the first autumn after my celiac diagnosis, the crisp apples gleaming golden and pink, their skins taut against crisp flesh, made me reach into my bags of gluten-free flour and start experimenting. I would not go the rest of my life without apple pie.

The secret to great pie dough is patience. Understand that gluten-free pie dough can be a little quick to wilt or turn tough. You really have to listen to it with your hands, with a deft touch and a pause before continuing on to the next step. Chill the dough for a long time, preferably overnight. You cannot eat the pie only an hour after imagining it, as you might be able to do with a typical pie. And sometimes, the dough will break apart into chunks, instead of rolling out neatly. Don't worry—just pick up the pieces and stitch them together with your fingers, pressing them into the pie plate to form the shape of a pie crust. No one will notice the little imperfections. The taste will reward you, fully.

And the apples? Those will always be gluten-free. Fill your gluten-free pie crust with apples that have been releasing their juices into sugar and allspice, steaming with cinnamon and flecked with vanilla bean, and you will be rewarded with a taste that makes your best friends moan and with the satisfaction of knowing you can make pie once again.

Gluten-Free Pie Crust

1½ cups sorghum flour
½ cup tapioca flour
3 tablespoons sweet rice flour
¼ teaspoon salt
3 teaspoons sugar
1 teaspoon strong cinnamon (I use Saigon cinnamon from World
    Spice Merchants)
8 tablespoons (1 stick) cold butter
1 large egg
2 tablespoons apple cider vinegar
¼ cup ice-cold water, or enough to make the dough stick
    together

Mixing the flours and butter. Using a stand mixer (or a food processor), combine all the dry ingredients. Cut the butter into little pieces, about ½ inch thick, and drop the pieces into the dry ingredients. Turn on the mixer again and mix on low speed until the butter has crumbled into pea-size pieces.

Adding the wet ingredients. Drop in the egg and apple cider vinegar as the mixer is running. Once they are incorporated, slowly drizzle the ice-cold water into the mixture, a little at a time, while the mixer is running. When the mixture coheres and looks like dough, turn off the mixer.

Refrigerating the dough. At this point, drop the ball of dough onto a large piece of parchment paper. (Prepare this ahead, unless you want to wipe dough off the box of parchment paper later!) Place another piece of parchment paper, the same size, on top of the dough. Gently, smoosh the dough outward, equally in all directions, until it is a thick, round cake of dough. Refrigerate the dough for as long as you can. Ideally, you should prepare the dough in the evening and refrigerate overnight. Take the dough out of the refrigerator at least 20 minutes before you want to work with it.

Preheating. Preheat the oven to 400 degrees F.

Rolling out the dough. Leave the dough in the parchment-paper sandwich and roll it out. By rolling it, gently, between the pieces of parchment paper, you will not need to add more flour to the mix. Roll it out to the size of the pie plate, then strip the top piece of parchment paper off the dough. Carefully, flip the dough into the pie plate. Using your fingers, gently press the dough outward, evenly, until you have extended it beyond the edges of the pie plate. You can crimp the edges at this point. If some of the dough falls off the sides, don't worry. Simply reattach the pieces to the crust-to-be by pressing in with your fingers. (Gluten-free pie crust is fragile, but it is also forgiving in the baking.)

Filling the pie crust. Fill the pie crust with the apple filling (recipe follows). Carefully cover the apple filling with another layer of pie crust. Pinch the edges to seal in the apples. Cut a small slit in the top crust to allow the steam from the cooking apples to escape. Put the pie in the oven. Bake for 15 minutes. Lower the oven's temperature to 350 degrees F and bake the pie for another 30 minutes. Check the pie sporadically to make sure the top is not browning too much. (If it is, cover the pie with some tin foil for the remaining baking time.)

Taking out the pie. The pie is done when you can insert a knife into the apples and have it move through them softly, when the crust is warm and golden, and when the juices from the apples are carmelizing along the edges of the crust. Take the pie out immediately when it has reached this stage. Cool for 20 minutes, then dig in.

Apple Pie Filling

8 apples, of various kinds (Honeycrisps, Jonagolds, Braeburns, and Granny Smiths)
1 cup sugar
1 vanilla bean
1 teaspoon strong cinnamon
1 teaspoon ground nutmeg
1 teaspoon allspice
juice of 1 lemon
splash of brandy or cognac

Slicing the apples. Peel the apples and core them. Slice them into solid slices—not so thin that they look like paper, and not so thick that you cannot wrap your mouth around them. Put all the slices into a large bowl.

Making the apple mixture. Cover the apples with the sugar and stir. Slice the vanilla bean down the middle and scrape out the paste from the inside of it. Put that paste in with the apples and sugar, then cut the shell of the vanilla bean into small strips and let those fall into the apples as well. Cover the apples with the cinnamon, nutmeg, allspice, lemon juice, and brandy. Stir well, making sure to coat each of the apple slices. Set the bowl aside to let the apples marinate in these juices for at least 2 hours before making the pie.

Feeds 8.

a sweet start to the new year

On New Year's Eve, as part of the three-course meal I made for myself, I grabbed the seven or eight Meyer lemons sitting on my drainboard, and I dabbled in some recipe creation. In the dead of winter, I desired sorbet—sweetness, with a hint of tartness, too.

A hybrid of the mandarin orange and the traditional lemon, first created in China, the Meyer lemon is a flash of brightness in the midst of dark winter. At a time when only a scant few fruits are blooming into season, the smooth-fleshed Meyer lemon arrives in time to remind us that there will be spring to come. On the West Coast, they arrive at farmers' markets and grocery stores in early November and stick around until February. After they leave, only one month remains of winter. After months of making Meyer lemon pie, or Meyer lemon simple syrup for teas, or Meyer lemon cream puffs (yes, they were gluten-free), I am sad to see them leave the markets. However, their disappearance means that the beginning of spring cannot be far away. And besides, there is always the next year.

Friends of mine, fellow bloggers in Northern California, have the audacity to complain that their Meyer lemon trees are so full and fertile that they have no idea what to do with all that fruit. Um, I wish I had that problem. I know what I would do. I would eat Meyer lemon sorbet every night, the way I did on New Year's Eve. Simple and elegant, this sorbet made the solitary evening feel more vibrant. It felt puckish with lemon, but not overpowering. In the lingering taste of the Meyer lemons was something mysterious. My tongue was tingling and asking for the answer to that mysterious taste. A hint of bergamot, perhaps?

The next afternoon, on New Year's Day, my friend Amal came over to help me celebrate the new year. We ate wild mushroom risotto, the way her Italian ex-mother-in-law-to-be had taught her to make it in Tuscany. For much of the meal, we discussed the complications of having an Italian ex-mother-in-law-to-be. We came to no answers, but the talking seemed to help. After our sumptuous risotto, I gave her a bowl of the Meyer lemon sorbet. She spooned some into her mouth, and then she grew quiet. After a moment, she said, quietly: "I don't even like ice cream. I haven't bought a pint since I returned to Seattle. But I love this." And then she grew quiet again, looking far away into the corners of the room. "This reminds me of walking with my grandmother in the afternoons, smelling her jasmine, being with her."

Nothing could have made me happier in that moment.

Meyer Lemon Sorbet

1 cup granulated sugar
1 cup Meyer lemon juice
1 egg white
zest of 1 Meyer lemon

Making the syrup. Heat the sugar and lemon juice together in a saucepan over medium-high heat. Watch the mixture carefully to make sure it does not boil over. (If you have a gas stove, you will have an easier time of maintaining an even heat. If you have an electric stove, be vigilant.) Keep a pastry brush in a glass of water next to the stove. As the liquids rise high in the pan, brush the insides of the pan with the wet pastry brush, which will prevent the sugar and lemon from burning on the sides of the pan. When the liquids have reached a temperature of 235 degrees on a candy thermometer, and the liquids have become a thickened syrup, remove the pan from the heat. Pour the syrup into a shallow dish. Place the dish in the refrigerator to cool to room temperature for at least 2 hours.

Preparing the sorbet. Beat the egg white in a stand mixer until it is frothy. Slowly drizzle the cooled syrup into the egg white and mix until well incorporated. Add the Meyer lemon zest. Stir until the zest is just mixed.

Put this liquid into your ice cream maker and let it run for about 15 to 20 minutes. If you take the sorbet out before it's completely hard, the taste will remain vivid. Transfer the sorbet into a freezer-safe dish and freeze to the desired hardness.

Feeds 2.

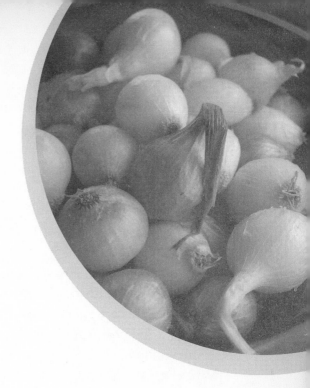

9

truly tasting my life

I had to nearly lose my life to write this chapter.

In the back of the ambulance, I kept falling out of consciousness. The medic shouted questions at me. "What is your name?" The urgency in his voice cut through the fog.

I didn't know my name.

I didn't know much of anything.

I knew that my arms and legs felt useless. At the best trauma hospital in Seattle, the nurses piled on eight or ten emergency blankets. Nothing stopped the trembling at the core of me. Deep under, I heard the urgent confusion in the nurse's voices—they wondered why they couldn't warm me up. From a great distance, a thought arose, "I'm dying." The thought vanished, along with any fear of it. My mind didn't have the energy to attach to it.

There was no struggle. No regret. There was no great epiphany, no white light. I was simply fading out.

In December 2003, my life spun around after I was hit by a

speeding white car. It could have been worse—people who saw my crumpled car were amazed that I survived at all. There was a terrifying day in the hospital, deep in shock and feeling close to death. Then, a year and a half of medical treatments, debilitating pain, and time for reflection.

Ample time for reflection.

Everything in our culture says we have to rush, to accomplish, to be better and bigger than everyone else. We don't know how to slow down. There's nothing like a near-death experience to make you stop rushing, and really live instead.

When you live with the knowledge, along your battered bones, that death could come at any moment, you live differently than you did before. You *live*. And you love every moment. The mundane feels miraculous.

When was the last time you felt the delicious thrill of being able to stand up straight while walking?

I will never forget the first time I could stand up straight after the car accident. It took me six weeks, six weeks of lying in a bed, then crawling to the bathroom, hobbled over and moving slowly to stop the sciatica pain from shooting down my leg. Somewhere in early February, I woke from my Vicodin sleep and walked to the shower. It felt like a victory in my body. The warm water surged on my back, and I could feel every drop on my skin. Afterward, I dried my hair, lifting my arms fully for the first time in weeks. When the weak winter sunlight broke through the clouds to enter my bathroom window, I smiled wide, and it did not hurt my head.

Deliberately, I grabbed my keys, nudged my toes into my slip-on shoes, and walked down the stairs to go outside for the first time in weeks. I walked toward the bakery, halfway down the block from my house.

(This was, of course, before I discovered that I should not be eating gluten. All the bread and pastries from that bakery, and the rest of my diet, turned out to be one of the reasons my injuries lingered for a year and a half. I know that now.)

The air felt damp on my cheek, and I started to cry. The pale fading-to-gray sky, the chipped paint on the crosswalk, the feeling of my feet walking evenly on the pavement—such joy.

When I walked into the bakery, fifteen minutes later—yes, it took me fifteen minutes to walk halfway down the block—my mind felt stuffed full of sensory experiences. How many times had I walked down that block and missed it all? The exact smell of exhaust from the bus. The ragged edges of the brick wall in front of the dry cleaner. The taste of sugared sweetness in the air ten feet in front of the bakery. The muted symphony of car horns, each car a different pitch. The sight of three small blackbirds on a telephone wire, huddled close together. In fifteen minutes, I had lived an entire life.

One step inside the bakery, and I had to close my eyes. The scents of cinnamon and yeast, chocolate and coffee, vanilla sugar and human bodies were so overpowering that I thought I would have to stop on the spot. Instead, I moved forward, slowly, gesturing for every new customer to go around me in their quest for immediate service. By the time I reached the counter, I knew what I needed. Nothing fancy. Just a cup of black coffee.

Claire, the young woman with the Victorian face, brown hair draped around her soft eyes, smiled and asked me where I had been. Everyone there knew me. Usually, I stopped in every afternoon. When I told her what had happened, her eyes grew pained. Before she could start her soothing apologies, however, I stopped her. "This has been the most remarkable six weeks of my life."

She poured the coffee in a white to-go cup, and I felt the warmth of it cupped between my hands. It felt enormously good.

I pulled out a twenty to pay for the coffee, and spontaneously, I made a decision. "Claire, keep the change. Whoever comes in next, let the change pay for their coffees, until the money runs out."

She stumbled. "What?"

"Walking here to buy this coffee was the best fifteen minutes of the last six weeks. I want everyone else to enjoy it, too." I waved and walked my slow dance home.

The next day, I walked back again. When I entered the bakery, Claire immediately said to me, "People were so pleased. Everyone said that you had made their day." I left there with tears in my eyes again.

In spite of all our defenses to the contrary, it is so easy to love people. We put up barriers, especially in thinking that we have to focus our energies on loving particular people. But after my car accident, I know differently.

Years ago, I sat in meditation on a retreat in the woods of Western Washington. We spent three days in silence, a group of strangers who knew each other's faces by heart by the end of the weekend. It is profoundly odd to not talk for three days. (No writing, either.) Somehow, the food tasted more vibrant than any food I had eaten before that. And it was, invariably, the simplest of hippie food: brown rice, sautéed vegetables, and salads. For many of the meals, I spooned little pools of tangy lemon-tahini dressing on top of my rice or greens. The taste of it—tart with the lemons; rich with the sesame depth of the tahini; smooth and filling—stayed with me through many a meditation session.

I wondered how the cooks made such simple food so beautiful. One day, toward the end of my time there, I took my dishes into the kitchen. And I saw, tacked above the stove, a simple sign: "The bigger the task, the more we have to slow down."

I have never forgotten that sign. Many a time, when I have been driving somewhere, worried I was going to be late, my mind flashed on that sign. And I remembered again, "This is the only time you are going to live this moment. Do you really want to experience it full of angst?" And so, I slowed down.

It might have saved my life a time or two.

We are, quite literally, what we eat. We gorge ourselves on bad fast food, go hours without eating for fear of gaining an ounce, and constantly doubt our own judgments about what to eat. No wonder we are all so overweight and running out of breath. We have forgotten the ineffable pleasure of simply eating.

And just what are we all running after? So many people eat frozen foods or takeaway from big-chain grocery stores, or make a three-minute pizza from a frozen gluten-free crust, a bottle of tomato sauce, and some previously shredded cheese. Okay, I understand the need to make dinner quickly, sometimes. But what are we gaining with all that saved time? What are we losing by not truly tasting our food?

Have you ever noticed how, in crowded grocery stores, people fidget, fitfully, in the long line they are standing in, their eyes darting right and left to see if the line on either side of them is moving just a little bit faster? They are back in traffic, desperate to get ahead. What would their lives be like if they relaxed their bodies and spent that time in line observing the human beings around them? Or stopped to take in all the smells of the grocery store? Or spent thirty seconds remembering how blessed they are to be stuck in a line with a cart full of food?

My dear friend Julie told me this story. Her mother, a dedicated and productive psychology professor at a university, was diagnosed with cancer. Her first thought was "Oh, good. Now I can slow down."

Do we need a death sentence to allow ourselves to truly taste our lives?

It has been through food that I have found the stillness I sought for years.

There's a little secret no one really tells you in cookbooks: when you cook with mindfulness and concentration, your food tastes better than when you rush. When we slow down to truly experience what is before us, the richness of life yields itself. When was the last time you leaned down toward the cutting board and took a deep whiff of fresh-cut ginger?

Before my celiac diagnosis, I bought roasted peppers in a jar when I felt like cooking something spicy. Now, I roast them myself, under the broiler. It takes five minutes and costs half the price of the jar. I taught myself how to make gluten-free truffle brownies, using rice flour and tapioca flour, and a 70 percent dark chocolate bar from France. Those brownies rose to chewy perfection. My god, the time I wasted ripping open a box of brownie mix and just adding an egg and water. Touched by human hands, made from scratch, and with slow attention—that food always tastes better than what is in packages.

There is something deeply meditative about kitchen tasks. The world can feel encroaching, sometimes coming apart at the seams. But take out an onion, peel it of its papery skin, watch it glisten in the light filtering through the window, and start to chop it into meticulous pieces. Within minutes, everything else has fallen away.

complex and saucy

What separates home cooking from fancy restaurant cuisine? An architectural presentation: an angular tower of matchstick apples, with pomegranate seeds falling toward the little dots of green pesto on a square white plate. When that arrives at the table of a restaurant, you feel like saying, "Ah. Now that I couldn't make at home."

Actually, we all could, with a little practice, but that's a different story.

In my mind, as well, there was something I savored at restaurants that seemed far beyond the ken of my stove—sauces. Food seems to taste better when it is arranged well, and better still when it is hovering above the surface of a little skim of brown sauce. As much as I admired the food I ate in my favorite restaurants, when I ate bread pudding in a pear sauce, or seared lamb chops surrounded by a mustard sauce, I grew a little depressed. "I'll never cook like this," I thought.

Nonsense.

Once I went gluten-free, and I thought I'd never eat in a restaurant again, I resolved to learn to cook sauces. Guess what? With a little patience, some mindful attention, and a willingness to learn, anyone who cares about food can learn to make a delicious sauce. My favorite chef in Seattle taught me how to make this one.

Red Wine Reduction Sauce

Wow your friends and family with your elevated cuisine by making this red wine sauce. It is the basis for coq au vin. Trail it over a square of grilled polenta for a visual feast. Lamb, beef, and sirloin—all are made better by a little red wine sauce.

        3 tablespoons high-quality olive oil
        1 carrot, peeled and diced
        ½ yellow onion, chopped
        2 stalks of celery, diced
        4 cloves garlic, peeled and smashed
        1 beefsteak tomato, quartered
        4 sprigs fresh thyme, chopped
        1 sprig fresh rosemary, chopped
        3 sprigs fresh sage, chopped
        4 cups red cooking wine
        2 quarts meat stock (chicken, beef, or veal stock will all do well
            here)
        1 tablespoon butter
        ½ teaspoon kosher salt
        ½ teaspoon cracked black pepper

Making the mirepoix. Bring a large stockpot to full heat. Add the olive oil. When the oil moves around the bottom of the pot as easily as water, add the carrots, onions, celery, and garlic to the pot. On medium-high heat, cook the vegetables, stirring occasionally, so as not to burn them. If you burn the garlic, begin again. Cook until the vegetables have caramelized, meaning they will have a rich, dark-brown color, about 10 minutes.

Adding the tomato and herbs. Add the tomato and fresh

herbs to the caramelized onions. When they become fragrant, after 1 to 2 minutes, add the red wine.

Reducing the liquid. Cook the vegetables, herbs, and red wine on medium heat until the volume of the wine has reduced by half, about 10 minutes. Keep on eye on the wine, stirring occasionally.

Cooking the sauce. When the wine has been reduced—perhaps 10 minutes—add the meat stock to the pot. Turn the heat to high and bring the mixture to a boil. Reduce the heat to medium. Cook the sauce until you have reduced this liquid by half its volume, 15 to 20 minutes.

Skimming the sauce. Throughout this entire process, skim the surface of the liquid for fat. Fat is the sauce's enemy. You won't ruin the sauce if you leave the fat on the surface, but the sauce will not be as clear, nor will it have as vivid a flavor. You don't want your sauce to taste like fat. So, skim the surface regularly.

Straining and finishing. When the liquid has reduced in volume by half, strain it through a fine-mesh sieve. Put the sauce back in the pot. Add the butter and whisk it in as it melts. Taste the sauce, then add the salt and pepper.

Serve with your favorite meat or vegetables and wow your guests.

Feeds 6.

dressing myself

When I was a kid, salad dressing only came one way: poured out of a bottle with a label on it. The blue cheese dressing glopped out of the jar with a solid plop. It didn't move; it didn't seem to come from a liquid. That white dressing with a blue cast just sat there, demanding to be spread across the iceberg lettuce. We ate more ounces of ranch dressing than is humanly decent to admit. And when my mother wanted to be fancy, we bought the Italian dressing. You know the one—it had little artificially colored bits of herbs floating in the viscous liquid.

In my twenties, I discovered balsamic vinegar, and then I thought I was sophisticated. I watched the little lava-lamp configurations of the dark vinegar swirl around the oil as I stirred it with a fork. A few cloves of garlic, a dollop of Dijon mustard, and I ate my greens like a good girl. So what if it tasted too much like the vinegar, and there were bites that seemed to be only oil? I felt virtuous for not buying my salad dressing from a bottle.

Champagne Vinaigrette

After I went gluten-free, I stopped buying any bottles of dressing. They were no longer viable for me. And unless I wanted to continue to eat vinegar-heavy salads, I had to learn how to make a proper vinaigrette.

Here it is.

¼ cup champagne vinegar
1 teaspoon Dijon mustard
1 teaspoon finely minced shallots
½ teaspoon kosher salt
½ teaspoon cracked black pepper
½ cup canola oil
¼ cup high-quality extra-virgin olive oil
¼ cup club soda

Preparing the vinaigrette. Put the champagne vinegar, Dijon mustard, shallots, salt, and pepper in a blender. Turn it on and mix well.

Emulsifying the vinaigrette. Slowly, drizzle the olive and canola oils into the blender as it runs. Blend for 1 full minute or more, after it is mixed. This will emulsify the vinaigrette, which means that the oils and vinegar will stick together. After the oils have emulsified, slowly pour in the club soda. This touch will make the vinaigrette taste subtler.

Storing the vinaigrette. If you make the vinaigrette in a blender, it will stay thick and mixed for weeks on end. Store it in a plastic squeeze bottle in your refrigerator.

Suggestions. You can use this method for any flavor of vinaigrette you choose: red wine vinegar; pomegranate champagne vinegar; tomato vinegar, and so on. Play with flavors and different oils to make your own favorite dressing.

Feeds 10.

well-stocked

Whenever Thanksgiving and Christmas came around, my mother went into a frenzy of planning. We all dreaded the day that we knew we could not avoid: the big shop. Mom made a huge list of everything she would need to make the holiday dinner: loaves of soft white bread for the stuffing, cream of chicken soup for the gravy, a giant turkey in a plastic bag, and a disposable roasting pan that buckled under the weight of the turkey as my mother lifted it into the oven.

Mostly, though, I remember unloading all the grocery bags when we returned home from the store. One entire bag was filled with cans of chicken broth. Whoever unloaded that bag stacked those cans neatly on the drainboard, sometimes in a pyramid like perky cheerleaders about to do flips. Throughout the feasting, my mother ordered one of us to use the hand-cranked can opener to pry open one can after another. The yellow fat globules that floated on the surface of the brown liquid always disgusted me. Of course, it was my job to hold the floating lid down into the liquid to strain the fat out of it, and then hand the can to my mother so she could make our gravy.

Oh, if only we had used homemade chicken stock.

It's so easy to make chicken stock. Before my celiac diagnosis, I thought this was something that only chefs could do. Now, I make a big pot of it every Sunday, and another one on Wednesday if I have made a lot of quinoa or soups.

Chicken Stock

The only requirement of chicken stock is that you stay home for four hours, listening to it simmer in the other room, as you slow down. Believe me, once you have made your first chicken stock, you will never open another can again.

1 fryer chicken, cut up into pieces (ask your butcher to do this for you)
3 yellow onions, chopped in half
3 large carrots, peeled and chopped roughly
4 ribs celery, washed and chopped roughly
1 head garlic, crushed
3 bay leaves
2 tablespoons black peppercorns
3 sprigs fresh rosemary
5 sprigs fresh thyme
½ bunch Italian parsley

Simmering the chicken. Put the chicken pieces into a large pot. Add enough cold water to cover the chicken by 2 inches. Bring the water to a boil. When it has boiled for 1 minute, turn the heat down to a simmer.

Skimming the water. Skim the surface of the water with a ladle to remove all the foam that arises. Let the water simmer for another 5 minutes and skim again. Pour the water and chicken through a colander. Put the chicken back in the pot.

Adding the flavorings. Add the onions, carrots, celery, and garlic to the pot and cover with cold water by 2 inches again. Bring to a boil. Turn down the heat. Add the bay leaves, black peppercorns, rosemary, thyme, and parsley to the stock. Bring to a boil again.

Simmering the stock. Turn down the heat to simmer the stock. Allow the stock to simmer for 3 to 4 hours. Do not stir. Leave it alone. You will know the stock is done when the smell is rich and flavorful and the broth is golden.

Straining the stock. Strain the stock and allow it to cool to room temperature. Put the strained stock in the refrigerator. It should last in the refrigerator for about 1 week. If you are not going to use it all in a week, freeze the stock. However, the stock will lose some of its flavor in the freezer. Besides, you're going to want to cook with it after you have made it!

Makes 2 quarts.

10

guilty
pleasures

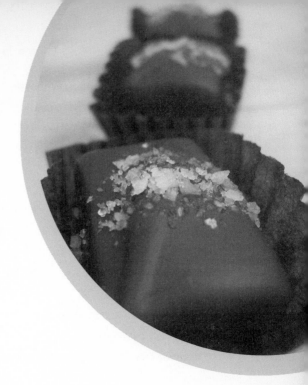

I have always loved food. My memory is redolent with smells of chocolate, baked potatoes with sour cream, barbecued steaks crispy from the grill, greasy fries that left salt on the tongue. Other people remember relatives, pets, or friends from childhood. I remember meals.

Christmas meant rich, buttery sugar cookies, slathered in frosting, gobbled from plates heaped high with goodies. Every Christmas morning we ate homemade sweet rolls with buttercream frosting. Christmas dinner meant the entire spread: turkey (I'd always steal hot mouthfuls of brown, crispy skin before we set the platter on the table), steaming mashed potatoes, canned cranberry sauce, and rolls covered in butter. After a few bloated hours of eyeing our new presents, we ate Mom's homemade pumpkin pie. We usually dipped our fingers in the bowl of whipped cream.

Summertime meant barbecues and potato salad. We woke up late and ate plates full of eggs and bacon or waffles straight out of the toaster. I ate bowl after bowl of sugary cereal, every few hours. My brother and I slipped into the pool in the late morning, swam to the side, then ran on the cement (our only act of daring for the day) to dive into the water, ferociously, slamming our toes down on the surface as we went in. We emerged from the chlorine to eat fried taquitos and bean dip from a can and every kind of chip known to modern man. Every night, we ate meat nearly as black as the charcoal beneath it.

Food flourished everywhere. And I never turned it down.

I was overweight for as long as I can remember. Pictures of me before kindergarten show a normal little girl, with spindly legs, a long neck, and a big grin. That doesn't seem like me. In my memory, I was always abnormal, swimming in extra flesh, awkward in my pudginess. I spent most of my life with my eyes facing downward, my shoulders slumped forward, my shirts untucked.

After I left my parents' house, I was not unhappy or lonely. But all throughout my twenties, I only glimpsed small glimmers—moments at a time, and no more—when I felt normal, in my weight, in my life. I carried far more baggage than the pounds society told me I needed to lose.

That baggage began to pile on in my childhood. My grandfather died when I was sixteen, while my family and I were living in England for the year. I rarely saw him, other than on tense vacations. Even when I did, he never really talked to me, since he suffered from shyness. But this I remember.

It was Christmastime; Granddad and I were sitting in the cramped living room. In the kitchen sat the empty papers of a quickly conquered Sees candy box. Grandma worked on dessert at the stove. I sat at a TV table watching a mindless program. Without thinking, I buttered a piece of French bread left over from dinner. I ate it quickly and then buttered another. Then another. Then another. Granddad looked on without saying a word. After my sixth piece, he turned toward me and said, "Don't you think it's time you stopped eating that bread?"

I ran to the bathroom and cried for an hour.

(Oh, if only someone had told me to stop eating the bread, for other reasons. What would my life—and the way I regarded my body—have been like if I had been diagnosed with celiac disease then?)

My seventeenth summer, I finally grew tired of feeling fat. I joined Weight Watchers. Every day of that summer, I biked the quarter mile to the downtown storefront, sandwiched between the health food store and the Wendy's fast food place. I sat among dozens of women, all of whom were much heavier than I, a fact I relished with secret glee. These sad shadows of flesh were all in their thirties, most had husbands and small children, and all of them carried a haunted expression. The Saturday weigh-in was a constant humiliation I carried with me all the rest of the days of the week. Would I lose a pound? Would I be that much closer to fitting in? The first week of the program, when I lived zealously on steamed broccoli and plain yogurt, I lost six pounds. Nothing had ever seemed better. Over the next two months, I continued to lose, although never anything approaching that sudden drop. When the summer had finished, I had lost a miraculous twenty-five pounds. I returned to school at the start of my senior year to compliments and jokes about my parents obviously not being able to feed me. But I quit Weight Watchers as soon as I started school again. The tragic confessionals of Saturday mornings depressed me. Women told stories of having to lock up ice cream from themselves, of measuring out ketchup by the teaspoonful, of begging their husbands to wait and see what they would look like once the weight disappeared. Many wept when they failed once again to lose an ounce on the gleaming silver scale. Going to those meetings made me feel even more like a sideshow freak than before. Other high school students had dates and car washes on Saturdays. I spent time at weight-loss centers.

When I was nineteen, after my freshman year in college and the typical diet of gulped burgers, fries, and too many pizzas, I had gained back the weight I had lost before senior year. And then some. Once again, I decided to deprive myself in a desperate measure to excise flesh. I ate fruit and tofu, cottage cheese, and dry toast. I weighed myself every morning, and most evenings, too. If the scale crept too high, even on hot days when Barbie dolls retained water, I drank large glasses of plain iced tea, one after the other, so the scale would slide down another pound. It was not uncommon for me to weigh myself seven or eight times a day. Every morning and every night, I ran laps around my backyard, too ashamed to jog on the streets where people could see me. As I pounded down the dirt with my tennis shoes, my knees aching at every step, the music blasting in my ears, I'd repeat my fat mantra over and over again: "I won't look like this anymore. I won't look like this anymore. I won't."

Everything started to ease when I hit thirty. Living in New York and traipsing the streets I had only dreamed of when I saw them in the movies—I learned who I was. I lost some weight with all the walking. When I lived with the wealthy family in London, I saw how much the wife agonized over the twenty pounds more that she weighed than the waiflike girls who walk around the streets of L.A. with enormous sunglasses covering their eyes. Seeing the sad absurdity of her struggle made me see mine more clearly. I ate great food, and I allowed myself to enjoy it. I grew up.

When I returned to Seattle after four years in New York, I came back home with a new knowledge of my body and a determination to eat well. I threw away all the junk food of my childhood and embraced olive oil and whole foods instead. Nothing fried. No more fast food. Ten servings of fruits and vegetables per day. I went to a fancy-schmancy gym and lifted weights, took African dance, worked out six days a week for an hour a day. I should have been the picture of health.

However, I couldn't lose weight. I did everything that every expert suggested I try, but that weight just wouldn't come off. The needle on the scale barely moved. I had surgery for a fibroid tumor in January 2003, which left me constantly enervated, no matter how well I ate.

I think now that is when celiac disease set in. Apparently, it can lie dormant for years, silently affecting us. A trauma to the body of some kind can kick it into action.

At the end of 2003, a white blur spun my car around, and I finished facing another way. Pain surged through me. I could barely walk. My back spasmed in time with my head.

So, two weeks later, I started a diet.

What?

That entire time is foggy in today's mind, so I cannot tell you why I thought it the best plan of action to start a popular diet for my New Year's resolution. Following a lifetime's tradition of regarding food as my enemy, I panicked. *I'm going to get fat.*

In my concussed head, I thought the best thing I could do for my body was to deprive it.

The worst night was when I writhed in such horrific pain from the sciatica shooting down my leg that I grew nauseated. No matter which way I shifted in the bed, I could not escape the electric fire shooting out from the small of my back. I cried. I tried to ignore it. I felt terribly alone. My stomach lurched with the pain and the trauma. Never one given to nausea, I had only thrown up twice in my life. That night made it three. Worse yet, I was so paralyzed by the pain and injury that I could not walk. I didn't make it to the bathroom.

My brother drove over from his house to help me. He cleaned up the carpet. He brought me some ginger ale. He brought me movies for the DVD player, so that I could stay in bed without feeling restless. Finally, he handed me a package of crackers, and told me, "You really need to nibble on these. It will help calm your stomach." I could feel the gaping acidic emptiness in my innards, and I knew that the crackers would soothe me. But in my mind, panic set in. "I'm not supposed to be eating carbs yet! That's not until next week!"

I spent the next year and a half in a pain-wracked body, just wishing for some energy, trying to avoid the wrong foods. If only I had known that those crackers were hurting me for a different reason than I believed.

And so I slipped back into the fear of food, the same way I had dived under the surface of our pool to blot out the noise of my parents yelling. The anxiety about what I ate? It was always chasing me. No longer a comfort, food threatened me.

In the spring of 2005, I was finally liberated from my abusive relationship with food. I was diagnosed with celiac disease.

Yes.

When my doctor told me that I had celiac disease, I said it out loud—yes!

Not the typical reaction, I know. Most people, when told they must live without gluten, begin grieving right away. Imagine being told that you cannot eat gluten again. When handed this news, most people shout, "No. No. No!" But I said yes.

My body had been battered and enfeebled before that diagnosis. Most of my friends and family, and perhaps some of the doctors, thought I was dying of a mystery disease. Within three days of cutting gluten out of my diet, I felt better than I had in two years. I rejoiced.

I could have easily grown depressed if I had focused solely on what I had to live without for the rest of my life. After all, an entire swath of the food world was suddenly closed to me. In my life before diagnosis, when I returned from traveling the world, I told friends about the meals I had eaten before I described the places I had stayed. Restaurants were my cathedrals, grocery stores my churches. And I loved bread, with a devotion most people save for Sunday services. Why was I not depressed?

Immediately, I could feel something lifting. Throughout my life, I had been haunted by food: drawn to it, yet eating it for the wrong reasons, most of the time. I ate fast, in mass quantities, when I was not hungry. Most of the time, I didn't even pay attention to my food.

When I was ten, I was devastated by a root beer float at a family gathering. When I saw that the melting vanilla ice cream supply was dwindling, I began eating my float as fast as I could, scooping spoonful after spoonful into my mouth in rapid fashion, my spoon clinking against the glass. There was only enough ice cream for a few of us to have seconds, and I wanted to be one of them. No, I needed to have seconds. However, as fast as I gulped, I could not beat my sixteen-year-old cousin, who casually gathered the last of the ice cream into his mug without even looking around. He did not know how much I suffered, not only because I couldn't have seconds, but also because I had not tasted my root beer float at all. In my urgent desire to have more, I hadn't enjoyed the first one.

Most of my life, that's how I ate. After I went gluten-free, however, something opened up in me. For the first time in my life, this truth shimmered within my gut: food is my path to healing.

Even a few bread crumbs can make me ill for three days. You would think that I would regard food as a poison. With all this hidden gluten, you would think I'd suspect every morsel of being a potential assassin. But I don't. In fact, it's the other way around now.

I had grown up restricted, living with fear as a force in the house. I knew, in my bones, what came of living by saying no—paralysis, misery, a tape loop worn thin for the numbers of time it has been played. Innately, I knew that I wanted more than a life of complaining and deprivation.

I wanted freedom.

I was not alone in having a bad relationship with food. Most Americans seem to regard food as an enemy. At group meetings, people talk about "trigger foods," the ones that open up the doors to the cavernous hole below, where they fall precipitously and eat to fill themselves up. Is food a shotgun, threatening to shoot them? Others eliminate entire food groups, as though they are little blue meanies ready to attack with pointy knives. People talk about carbohydrates as though they are the devil.

Well, for me, some carbohydrates are, such as wheat, rye, barley, triticale, or spelt.

I have this theory. I think the reason all these no-carb/low-carb diets have been so popular is that undiagnosed celiacs have tried them and felt mysteriously better. They didn't know why, but they just felt lighter. And so they stayed with these overly rigid programs, thinking that was the cause of peace. Instead, it was the lack of gluten.

Emotional eating overwhelms many of us. When we talk about comfort foods, we aren't talking about the comfort of a warm blanket on a cold night, or the feeling of someone else's legs entangled with ours in bed. We are talking about feeding ourselves, almost in a frenzy, to stave off feelings with food. I did that, too. I used food as a defense, as a layer against the world, as a muffling of the loud noises in my mind. On those days, I ate a lot of macaroni and cheese from a box, an entire bag of potato chips, and some ice cream sandwiches. Truly, I never really tasted them.

After I realized that I could never eat gluten again, I slowed down. Being forced to make everything from scratch made me take the time to truly experience my food. Keeping a food blog meant that I stopped to take photographs of the meals I made before I took a bite. Looking at the food through a camera lens was a way of honoring what I ate, noticing the beauty in it, instead of scarfing it down immediately. When I started hearing back from readers, saying they were making dinners for their families, based on what I had written about the week before, I took even more care in the preparation of my food. I was developing an entirely new relationship with food.

My world expanded. I began to love food in a way I never could have imagined when I was younger.

Now that I am living definitively gluten-free, I realize that it took about six months for my intestines to heal, fully. That's the remarkable thing: all that healing came through food.

I really feel as though I am a self I have never known before.

Finally, I have the boundless, happy feeling of exercise. In the afternoons, I bike the Burke-Gilman trail or roller-blade around Greenlake, singing as I go. Most evenings, I am bobbing in the pool or walking around my neighborhood. On the weekends, I glide along Lake Union in a kayak or take late-afternoon yoga classes. It turns out that it was the gluten that kept me on the couch every afternoon, for years, wanting to be well but not able to move.

The exercise also triggered another shift. My body changed. I began losing weight, dropping dress sizes, wearing tank tops in the summer. Without dieting or ever weighing myself, I began having the body I always wanted. I'm still not a size two, or even a size six, but I am strong and healthy and alive. For the first time in my life, I love being in my body.

It's not that I'm eating any less food. In fact, I probably eat more. I sample all the foods I create for my Web site, and I do more than nibble. If it is gluten-free, I try it. Knowing that I am writing about food, and wanting to give my body the food that will nourish my health, colleagues and friends give me food for every holiday and birthday. And yet, in spite of that, the weight I've carried around all my life started to fall off me, without me trying. Why?

More and more research is showing that the traditional definition of celiac disease is far too narrow. In the past, you were diagnosed with celiac disease only if you had terrible diarrhea and couldn't put on weight. But now, studies are showing that some people with celiac disease can't lose weight. No matter how hard they work or try to diet, the weight just stays on. It's a function of the damaged small intestine, the way that individual's body reacts to gluten. Deprived of nourishment, the body craves more and more food, in a desperate attempt to get some vitamins and minerals, protein and fiber. Many of us overeat not because we are weak or mindless but because we are trying to keep our bodies alive. We don't know it, of course, and so we blame ourselves for not being able to lose weight. And then we reach for another box of cookies, full of gluten.

Once I was diagnosed, I lost those mindless, desperate cravings. Instead, I simply ate my food and celebrated when my body felt good.

It went deeper than that for me, as the months continued. The better I felt, the more I realized that I had never allowed myself to truly taste my food before. Every bite arrived with a dash of guilt, a pinch of regret, and a spoonful of numbness. Every time I ate, it sounded like, *You shouldn't.* Or, *That has way too many calories, and now you'll never get a boyfriend.* Or, *Hurry up and eat. Get more.* I know I am not the only one who has eaten like this. Isn't this most of us? We are so confused as to what causes cancer or makes us put on weight or increases the chance of premature wrinkles that we regard every bite as suspect. There is so little joy in the way we eat food in this country.

So as soon as I started feeling better and regaining my energy, I made a daring decision. Since food was my means to healing, I decided to enjoy every bite of food I ate. I chewed with a happy mouth. I chose steaks on occasion, and I relished the chance to taste the dense chewiness of the meat and the explosion of rich saltiness in that one bite of grilled fat along the edge. Whatever my body desired—not my fast brain, the one that panted, in a rush, for famil- iar old foods, but my gut—I ate it. Oh sure, there was the month, early on, when I was so delighted to find gluten-free foods in the grocery store that I bought everything with that label. Gluten-free does not mean calorie-free. But I knew that I would grow tired of eating packaged cookies and pancake mixes. I did. After a couple months, I found out from listening to my body that what I wanted most often was fresh fruits and vegetables, gluten-free grains, and foods made from scratch. By following the lead of my healing body, I began eating the way every nutritionist recommends. Yes, there were the fingerling potatoes roasted in duck fat for Christmas, and they were amazing. But most days, what I want is some quinoa sim- mered in homemade chicken stock, and a big green salad with goat cheese.

When food is an elixir, a joyful, sensory experience—and espe- cially when it's the path to health—I don't eat too much of it. Add the laughter of friends ringing in your ears as you cook it, and you have one of the central pleasures of life. That food, I taste, fully. And then I'm full, quickly.

I have finally learned how to trust my body.

However, sometimes you still just need some macaroni and cheese.

As I write this book, it is winter, one day past the shortest day of the year. The sun sets in Seattle at 4:22 in the afternoon. This is an improvement over a few days ago, but only by a few slivers of sunlight. It's dark. It's cold. Last week, we had a tremendous windstorm that left half of the Puget Sound area without power for a week. I'm lucky because my house never lost power. However, the air coming in along the sides of the windows is chilly. Our bodies want to hibernate in this weather, but we still keep driving ourselves. What does my body crave?

Starches. I want some macaroni and cheese.

There's nothing wrong, inherently, with the starchy, salty, rich foods in life. In fact, they can be an enormous pleasure. My problem, before, was eating them with mindless abandon, buying them in a package and having them in my stomach within three minutes. No bag of french fries will ever make me feel less lonely. Fast-food fried chicken is not going to help me finish that project. (Besides, it would leave greasy fingerprints on the keyboard.) Chocolate-chip cookies from the refrigerated section of the store—wrapper ripped off and the log of dough cut into slices—just won't do your taxes for you.

However, if I choose that food, that's a different story. Since I have to make everything from scratch, there are no impulse binges on comfort food anymore. Now, making macaroni and cheese is a ritual, complete with white sauce, slowly stirred, and a small pile of Spanish sheep cheese. By the time I have shopped for the fresh ingredients, come home and cooked them, waited for the dish to bubble and brown within my oven, and taken a photograph of the finished product, I only need a small bowl to satisfy me.

The comfort of knowing that I can eat the good food I choose—and be healthy—makes me happy. I'm not held hostage by my food anymore. I choose it.

That is true freedom.

a new twist on an old dish

One evening in late winter, I came home from school in the dying golden light, possessed by an idea. My eleventh graders and I had been discussing *Their Eyes Were Watching God,* and in particular the scene in which Tea Cake takes Janie's $200 and throws a huge feast for the town. What did he provide? Fried chicken and macaroni and cheese. Simply discussing the scene made everyone in the room hungry. Walking away from school, I felt a keen hunger for macaroni and cheese, followed by a sharp moment of grief that I could not make it.

Before my celiac diagnosis, I often had packages of frozen macaroni and cheese in the house. Slip it in the microwave and in five minutes flat it was in my hands, bubbling hot. But that's just it— flat. The taste was always the same. It was never mine.

In the first six months after my celiac diagnosis, I had been dancing in the kitchen, experimenting with tastes. My first impulse was to cook foods that naturally did not contain gluten. Pizza, and pies, and pasta? Bah. Who needed them?

But that evening, coming home after school, I realized that I had turned a corner. Suddenly, I did not want to go the rest of my life without eating macaroni and cheese. I needed to make some.

That night, as I grated and stirred and folded, I remembered the feeling of being a kid. Of desperately wishing that I could be in my own kitchen, as an adult, making macaroni and cheese for myself. And the wished-for adult remembered that kid, and appreciated her kitchen, with the golden light falling through the windows, even more.

God, that macaroni and cheese tasted good.

Macaroni and Cheese

I package gluten-free pasta
4 ounces unsalted butter
4 ounces white rice flour
4 cups whole milk
pinch of nutmeg

2 cups grated cheese (try Manchego, but any good goat or
    sheep cheese will do)
½ teaspoon kosher salt
½ teaspoon cracked black pepper
½ cup gluten-free bread crumbs

Preheating. Preheat the oven to 450 degrees F.

Cooking the pasta. Cook the gluten-free pasta according to the manufacturer's directions. Drain and set aside.

Making the roux. In a saucepan over medium heat, melt the butter completely. Stir in the rice flour with a big spoon and cook for 3 to 4 minutes, stirring continuously until the flour is cooked. This loose ball of dough is called roux. Set the roux aside.

Making the cheese sauce. Put the milk in a saucepan with a pinch of nutmeg. Bring to a boil. As soon as the milk begins to boil, add bits of the roux to the milk, about 2 tablespoons at a time. Whisk the milk and roux together. The sauce will begin to thicken after 3 to 4 minutes. Add more of the roux, in the same amount as before. Whisk continuously and watch it thicken. Repeat this process until you have incorporated all of the roux into the milk. Add 1 cup of the grated cheese into the thickening sauce. Continue whisking. Add the salt and pepper. Taste the sauce to make sure it works for you.

Baking the macaroni and cheese. Toss the pasta into the cheese sauce. Stir it around, then pour into an oiled baking dish. Top the pasta and sauce with the rest of the cheese and bread crumbs. Bake in the preheated oven for 15 to 20 minutes, or until the top is well-browned.

Feeds 4.

finger-lickin' good
and gluten-free

I'm not the most sophisticated cook in the world. I adore food, in all its natural forms, and I have so much to learn. So much. I have a gourmet taste, on a modest budget, and more enthusiasm than art for it. But still, most people stand astonished in my kitchen. We have become an entire nation of people who long to make our own food, yet we don't know how to do it.

So people eat crappy fried chicken, desperate for some taste in the cardboard and chemicals, and eat more, because there's only so much taste in chicken wilting under heat lamps in the grocery store—or worse yet, at the fast-food chain, where the grease smell assaults me as I drive by it. And then they worry that they are growing fat, and massively at risk of a heart attack, and life still doesn't taste as good as they had hoped. *I know*, they think, *maybe if I had lower-fat chicken, I could eat more of it. And finally, I will be filled up.*

Have you ever noticed that home-cooked food fills you more than any takeout ever could? And when you really, truly taste it, you eat far less than of the junk?

I remember the taste of the best fried chicken I have ever eaten. My mother made it, about fifteen years ago. I had graduated from college, and my brother was just behind me. He invited one of his best friends home for dinner, and I came over, too. My mother worked all day, coating the chicken in peppery flour and frying it in batches, whipping mashed potatoes, making gravy from scratch, and baking homemade biscuits. At this point in her life, she made more food from scratch than from a package, which was a shift from my childhood. Still, this was a special occasion, and it took her several hours. The table was laid out with napkins and wine glasses. We all sat down to eat. Matt, my brother's friend, dug in. From the first moment he started eating, he looked stricken, not with pain but with pleasure. His face melted into a smear of happiness. As he grew more and more ecstatic with the taste of the chicken, he finally just had to do it—he groaned. He groaned and hit his fist against the edge of the table, in an animal grunt that expressed for all of us the way that chicken tasted. My mother grinned.

That's what we're longing for—that entire experience—not some fish-slurry-covered-half-the-fat-and-what-the-hell-is-really-in-it chicken.

After all, there's nothing like homemade fried chicken, dredged in gluten-free flour, juicy and peppery, shared with friends.

Fried Chicken

1 fryer chicken, about 4 pounds, cut up into pieces (ask your
    butcher to do this)
1 quart buttermilk
2 tablespoons kosher salt
2 tablespoons cracked black pepper
4 cups canola oil
4 eggs
¼ cup milk
1 cup sorghum flour
1 cup rice flour
3 cups gluten-free bread crumbs

Soaking the chicken. Using a large bowl, soak all the chicken
pieces in the buttermilk. Let them marinate overnight.

The next day, remove the chicken pieces from the buttermilk. Pat them dry with paper towels. Season all the pieces
with salt and pepper, coating all the sides.

Preparing the oil. Put a 12-inch skillet on the stove. Add the
canola oil, which should come up to ½-inch deep in the skillet.
Turn the burner on high and heat the oil until it is 350 degrees F.

Coating the chicken. Whisk the eggs and milk together
until combined. Set up the breading station: a saucer with
the sorghum and rice flours combined, a bowl with the egg
mixture, and a saucer with the gluten-free bread crumbs. With
your left hand, dredge a chicken piece in the flour mixture to
coat evenly. Shake off the excess flour. Dunk the chicken piece
into the egg mixture with your left hand. Coat the chicken in
the egg mixture, using your right hand, until it is thoroughly
coated. Remove the chicken and place it onto the saucer with
the bread crumbs. With your left hand, coat the chicken with
the bread crumbs. This way, your left hand stays dry, and your
right hand will be the wet hand. Repeat this with all the chicken
pieces and place them on a waiting plate.

Frying the chicken. Once the oil is 350 degrees F on your
thermometer, carefully add the chicken pieces into the skillet

and turn the heat down to medium-high. Cook the chicken until the side that is in the oil is browned, which should be about 5 minutes. Turn the chicken pieces over. At this point, the oil should be maintained at 250 to 300 degrees F. If the oil dips below that temperature, turn the heat to high. Cook for another 10 to 12 minutes, or until the breast pieces reach an internal temperature of 160 degrees F and the legs reach an internal temperature of 180 degrees as noted on a meat thermometer.

Finishing the chicken. Put a wire rack above a large pan. Take out the chicken pieces from the skillet and place them on the wire rack, allowing the excess grease to drain into the pan below. Eat the chicken with delight.

Feeds 4.

sometimes, i still need a slice

The best evenings were when we found out we were going to Shakey's, for sizzling-hot pizzas delivered to our table, with the sound of pinball machines—and later Ms. Pac-Man and Frogger— surrounding us as we ate. Maybe we had just finished a big soccer game, or my parents couldn't stand another night in the house. Either way, I was happy. The thin crust crackled when I bit it, slightly burnt at the edges. I loved the stamped-out pepperonis and the little greasy crumbles of sausage, evenly brown, and filled with fat. I ate my fair share of that.

It didn't seem to matter just how bad the pizza was. I loved the cheesy goodness. Eventually, I did have to draw the line at the pizza from the lunchroom at my high school, which came in soggy squares and so much oil on the top that we had to wipe it off with paper napkins, which immediately became transparent from the amount of fat they soaked up. This is the place that also served us french fries so greasy we could actually wring them out like dishcloths.

When I grew into adulthood, I ate increasingly great pizzas. Some were deeply memorable, like the thin-crust, hot-from-the-oven slice

I ate in Florence, Italy, just off the Piazza Santa della Croce. I was there alone for the weekend, not knowing a word of Italian, in the middle of February, when there were no other tourists. But I could point to a slice and smile. This slice restored me to myself: the bite of the garlic; the supple depth of the tomato sauce; the fresh mozzarella, better than any I had ever tasted. I sat at a table by myself, outside the café, waiting for a hailstorm to stop, looking out over the piazza, eating my pizza, utterly at peace.

Finally, there were the thousand gorgeous slices of pizza I ate at Sal and Carmine's, on 101st and Broadway, just across the street from my apartment building in Manhattan. Coming home after a long day of exploring, writing, and gallivanting, I'd emerge from the subway at 103rd Street. If the air biting at my hands and cheeks felt particularly cruel, I'd have to stop in for a hot slice before I ducked into my building and ascended the elevator to my apartment. A long sliver of a store, with little-to-no decoration, Sal and Carmine's was only there to sell pizzas. Slices, mostly. I'd order one (or two) cheese slices and wait. With this pizza, I was perfectly content with merely cheese. Sal (or Carmine; I couldn't keep them straight) grunted hello, then turned toward the large ovens, and expertly slid out my slice and slipped it onto a white paper plate. He'd smack the paper bag with a flick of his wrist, for clearly the five thousandth time, and it would make a satisfying pop as it opened to the room. Then, he'd slide in my slice and hand it to me. I'd open the bag again to sprinkle red pepper all over it and throw in a couple of napkins. He'd slide me a Dr. Brown's root beer, and I'd wave good-bye. Sometimes, I'd even wait until I'd crossed the street before I'd take a bite. But most of the time, I'd walk across Broadway with an enormous slice of pizza, folded over, hovering above my mouth.

When I first found out I couldn't eat gluten, I knew that I'd be fine, because I didn't want to be that sick, ever again. But what about pizza? I thought I'd never eat it again.

But I don't give up that easily.

With rustic crusts, and a plethora of good gluten-free pizza mixes on the market, those of us who eat gluten-free can still eat pizza.

Instead, I moved on, with a mind full of memories, and the persistence of invention, until I found a gluten-free pizza crust that works for me. Eventually, those mouths full of basil and spicy sauce will join the memories of Florence and Chicago and the median at 101st in the darkness. I'll no longer think of it as only gluten-free pizza. Eventually, it will just become pizza.

Pizza Dough

2¼ teaspoons active dry yeast
1 teaspoon sugar
½ cup warm water
1 cup sorghum flour
1 cup white rice flour
1 cup tapioca flour
½ cup potato starch
1 teaspoon baking soda
1 teaspoon salt
2 teaspoons xanthan gum
1 egg
1 teaspoon apple cider vinegar
4 tablespoons high-quality extra-virgin olive oil
¼ to ½ cup club soda at room temperature
handful of cornmeal

Activating the yeast. Combine the yeast, sugar, and warm water in a large bowl and mix gently. Set aside until the mixture has combined and swelled to twice its size, which should take about 15 minutes.

Preheating. Preheat the oven to 200 degrees F.

Combining the dry ingredients. Put the sorghum flour, white rice flour, tapioca flour, and potato starch into the bowl of the stand mixer. Combine. Add the baking soda, salt, and xanthan gum. Combine well.

Adding the liquid ingredients. While the stand mixer is running, add the yeasty water, the egg and apple cider vinegar, and then 3 tablespoons of the olive oil. Allow the mixer to beat these liquids into the dry ingredients on low speed. Pour in the club soda in a slow drizzle. Pour in only as much as is needed to wet all the ingredients completely. The dough should feel soft and firm, like a baby's bottom. Turn off the oven.

Kneading the dough. Attach the dough hook to the mixer and stir the dough on medium speed for 5 minutes. This will give the dough a chance to cohere more evenly. It will also whip air into the dough, which will cut the usual density of gluten-free bread. After 5 minutes, turn off the mixer and transfer the dough to an oiled bowl. (If you do not have a stand mixer, knead the bread by hand on a gluten-free-floured surface for at least 10 minutes.)

Allowing the dough to rise. Put the bowl into the oven, with a damp towel over the top of it. Leave the bowl there for 90 minutes. The dough will not have risen much at this point. There is no gluten to stimulate rising. Accept that.

Baking the pizza dough. Take the bowl out of the oven and turn the oven up to 450 degrees F. Sprinkle a handful of cornmeal onto a pizza tray or a baking sheet. Place the pizza dough onto the tray and start to slowly spread the dough to the outer edges of the tray with your hands. Work gently, with the heel of your hands. When the dough has reached the edges of the tray, smooth the edges with your fingers. Let the dough rest for 20 minutes. Then, sprinkle the remaining olive oil on the surface of the dough. Slide the tray into the oven and bake for 7 minutes, or until the top is browning and the olive oil has been absorbed.

Topping the pizza. Top the pizza with your favorite sauce or vegetables, meats, and cheeses. Slide the tray into the oven again and bake for 10 minutes or so, until the cheese has melted and the sauce is bubbling.

Suggestions. There are, of course, a hundred different ways to top pizza. I'm especially fond of fresh mozzarella, basil, goat cheese, artichoke hearts, and prosciutto. Feel free to play with the flour combinations in this recipe, which is only a guide. I rarely make the same one twice.

Feeds 4.

those fig cookies you remember, but better

As an adult, I've lost my taste for enriched white flour, everything stuffed with sugar, and anything wrapped in plastic. Before my celiac diagnosis, I never knew what *good* felt like. Now that I know that my enervation and headaches were directly related to the evil gluten, I don't miss the stuff.

Except, sometimes, in the winter, I miss Fig Newtons.

I don't know why, exactly. All of them are the same size, the cookie part is a bit dry, and the fig is a uniform shape, ending at the edge. But when I was a kid, I grabbed stacks of them from the rattly plastic tray and ate them while reading my favorite books. Maybe it's something about the dark wintertime—the holidays over, the rain incessant— that makes me want to curl up with a book and some cookies.

So what could I do? I had to make up a recipe for gluten-free fig cookies.

After months of relying on gluten-free flour mixes, I finally took the plunge and started experimenting with all the alternative flours sold in little bags. And now I know them all so well that I just reach for them and start making up a recipe without needing to consult books. I just start baking.

That old feeling under my hands: the patting reassurance of baking without trepidation. Warm butter, creamed sugar, the sharp tug of nutmeg in my nose. The lovely, soft pull of dough. And that intoxicating aroma as the sweet, spicy cookies are baking in the oven.

These cookies taste familiar and exotic at the same time. The thick fig spread tastes like the stuff we ate as kids but with an adult twist—a liberal spilling of port. The dark brightness, the sticky consistency, and the little flecks of fig seeds all make these a joy to eat. Bite down and taste the molasses and nutmeg cookie crumble in your mouth, and then dart your tongue around to lick the fig off your teeth. They're milk-dunkable and sophisticated at the same time. I dare you to eat just one.

I hope these help you feel like a kid again.

Fig Cookies

Fig Spread
(to be made at least 24 hours in advance of the cookies)

> ½ pound of dried figs (I use light brown Calimyrna and dark Mission figs)
> ½ cup pomegranate juice
> ¼ cup port
> ¼ cup Meyer lemon juice (or ¼ cup lemon juice with 1 tablespoon sugar)

Preparing the fig spread. Chop the figs into quarters. Put the pieces into a large bowl and cover with the liquids. Soak the figs for at least 24 hours. Before you make the cookies, drain the figs of the liquid, except for a few tablespoons. Put the figs and remaining liquid in a food processor and blend to make a thick paste, somewhat like a tapenade consistency.

Fig Cookie Dough

> 1 cup brown rice flour
> 1 cup sorghum flour
> ½ cup tapioca flour
> ½ teaspoon baking soda
> 1 teaspoon baking powder
> ½ teaspoon xanthan gum
> 1 teaspoon salt
> 2 teaspoons fresh ground nutmeg
> ½ cup packed brown sugar
> ½ cup unsalted butter, softened
> ½ cup organic cane sugar (this is key, because it has a granular consistency)
> 1 large egg
> 1 teaspoon vanilla
> 2 tablespoons molasses

Preparing. Preheat the oven to 350 degrees F.
Combining the dry ingredients. Mix all of the dry ingredients in a medium-size bowl. Set aside.

Creaming the butter and sugar. Put the softened butter into a mixer (if you don't have a stand mixer, you really should splurge on one. It makes all the difference in the world). Add the brown sugar and organic cane sugar to the butter and cream together. Cream only until well blended, then turn off the mixer.

Finishing the dough. Add the egg, vanilla, and molasses. Mix until just blended. Add the dry ingredients and mix until thoroughly blended.

Refrigerating the dough. Refrigerate the dough in the refrigerator for at least 1 hour. This is key with gluten-free doughs.

Rolling out the dough. After you have chilled the dough, roll out half the dough to a 1-inch thickness. (Be sure to flour the board with gluten-free flour and be patient. Gluten-free dough can be hard to roll.) Lay this dough onto a baking sheet that is covered with parchment paper or a Silpat. Slather the fig spread over the surface of the dough, stopping about one inch from the edges. Roll out the rest of the dough and lay it over the fig spread. Crimp the edges to seal in the fig spread.

Baking the cookies. Slide the baking sheet into the oven for 15 minutes, checking occasionally to make sure the cookies aren't browning too much. Take the cookies out of the oven when they are firm to the touch and just starting to brown. Let them cool on a wire rack for 10 minutes.

Cutting the cookies. When the cookies have cooled slightly, cut the edges off to make even lines. (Don't throw them away! These are delicious, too.) Slice the giant cookie into small squares, and they will look like those fig cookies of your youth.

Makes 30 cookies.

11

feeling comfortable in the kitchen

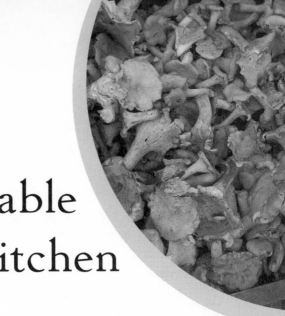

Having to go gluten-free turned me into a gourmet.

I can no longer rely on prepackaged food, even if it is labeled gluten-free. Don't misunderstand—I'm thrilled that gluten-free crackers, pretzels, energy bars, and cereals exist. They're good in-between foods for me. But for my main meals? I want every taste to be exquisite. Singular. Extraordinary. I want to taste something different every day. I want to taste the world. So, instead of examining the labels on packages, scrutinizing them to see if I can eat them, I search out high-quality whole foods that are naturally gluten-free. Locally caught salmon. Asparagus in May. Peaches in late July. French lentils. Truffle oil. Triple cream cheese. More, every day, more. Then, I cook. I throw tastes around the skillet and dance in the kitchen and sing for my supper, just to see what emerges.

I eat well.

Friends call to say, "Hey, what have you been up to?

"Cooking," I say. "Oh, and writing."

And then I start gushing about Spanish olive oils and sea salt from

Venice. I tell them about the chocolates from France I just tried. Or, I tell them about my escapades with making gluten-free ravioli. They laugh, a little, because of the enthusiasm in my voice. But they all want to come over for dinner.

I love the process of cooking. I love the smells that arise from below me as I cut and sliver and sauté. I love the sight of a knife slicing into a tomato, a leek starting to soften in a skillet, a soft cheese clinging to the spoon that holds it. I love the sounds: sizzling, dripping, splattering, burbling. I love the texture of silky olive oil on the tongue and the rough-hewn feeling of meat crumbled into a pan. And the tastes? Oh, the tastes.

Since my celiac diagnosis, I have been chopping meditatively, rocking my knife through winter vegetables and waiting for the spring to eat fresh fruit again. Cooking has become so deep a part of my day—a place without words, primal and alive—that by 4 P.M., when I'm headed home from work, my fingers actually start itching to be in the kitchen again. Whether it is cluttered or clean, my kitchen makes me happy. It's where I can play, where I can create. Home for the day, I crank up the CD player and sing as I slap together something new. Sautéed halibut with green-olive relish. Jamaican jerk chicken. A black bean salad with mango salsa and avocado. Butternut squash soup, with rosemary and smoked paprika. What will I try next? I don't know. It's always an adventure. Usually, I decide when I find something at the farmers' market that day.

Of course, the fact that I broadcast my meals via photographs and recipes on my Web site pushes me to cook every night. As people wrote to me, thanking me for gluten-free recipes that took only moments to make and tasted great, I found more of an incentive to cook and create. This wasn't just about me any longer. I was no longer alone in my kitchen.

I used to feel as though I should clear an afternoon to make that cake or casserole. However, after I stopped eating gluten, I have cooked a new meal—often inventing the recipe—at least four times a week. Every time, I am surprised by how little time and energy it takes. In fact, cooking rejuvenates me. I gain so much more from those twenty minutes or two hours of cooking than I would have by driving to the store and buying something in the gourmet deli section. Everything tastes so much better when I cook it at home.

I cannot imagine a better evening than one in which I'm standing at the stove, laughing with someone I love nearby, as we wait to eat, inhaling the smells of food together. At the end of the evening, I am sated and ready for more the next day. Flopping on the couch with leftovers could never make me this happy.

From structure comes freedom. If I had not been told that I had to live gluten-free, I never would have found the freedom of cooking. I never would have found myself so firmly planted in my kitchen. And all is right with the world in my kitchen.

So come on, everyone. For all those of you who claim you have no time to cook at home: stop talking and start cooking.

some guidelines for how to be comfortable in the kitchen

My students are always astonished to hear the first rule of my classroom: you are human beings before you are students. What do I mean by that? They are individuals, fascinating and complex, with enormous lives outside the confines of my classroom. I spend fifty minutes a day with them; I can teach them only so much. Besides that, what I want them to know is this: instead of trying to fit themselves into the rules of good writing, I want them to bring themselves into the process. I want them to relax; to learn how to trust the physical act of their pens moving across the page; to play; to allow themselves to make mistakes; to revise and revise, all of it in the spirit of learning, rather than trying to be right.

Along with this, I have always said: I'm not an expert at this. Sure, I've been writing, seriously, for twenty years, and I've been teaching writing for ten years. But mostly, like you, I'm someone who is continuously learning. I'm still practicing, and I always will be. I'm not done; I'm just a little bit farther ahead on the path. Let me point out a way for you.

They always seem grateful. They tell stories and laugh and feel comfortable enough to write every day. And mostly, they all become better writers.

These guidelines are presented in the same spirit. I'm no expert in the kitchen, yet. But what I lack in culinary school training, I make up for in exuberance and patience. Learning to live in the kitchen, according to the following guidelines, helped me to create a life filled with great food and laughter. I hope these guidelines will do the same for you.

play with your food

"Don't play with your food!" parents across the country cry out at the dinner table.

But really—why not?

Without the joy of playing with our food, we could never learn what we like. Food should be savored, not simply chewed. One of the ways I became a better cook over the course of my life—and particularly after I stopped eating gluten—was by listening to my insatiable curiosity. I will try anything now, as long as it does not have gluten. I will never forget the first time I tasted sushi, when I was a teenager. The idea of raw fish? Oh no. But the easy, meaty chew of tuna? Fantastic. If I had been safe and stuck to what I knew, I would never have experienced what is now an essential taste. I shudder to think how narrow my world could have been, if I hadn't learned to play with my food.

My young nephew, Elliott, adores all kinds of "strange" foods. He eats quinoa, steamed kale, and garlic mashed potatoes with gusto. I would like to think I play some part in this, since I taught him the sniffing game.

When he was just a little over one, I was babysitting him for the entire day. By the late afternoon, I had nearly run out of activities, and I was about to resort to a DVD. However, when I passed through the pantry, an idea arose. "Hey, Elliott! Let's sniff some of these foods." I pulled up a chair and then sat him on my lap.

Together, we gazed up at the shelves of foods before us. He pointed to one—brown sugar, in the first instance—asked me to tell him the name, and then dove his nose into it. That first day, he couldn't really sniff properly. He'd gush air out, instead of in, and he clearly didn't smell much. But somehow, the smell of cocoa powder penetrated, and his eyes grew wide. He took a long whiff, then went back for more, nodding several times before saying, "Smells pretty sweet!" He was hooked.

We have to sniff during every visit, now. For months, his interest in sniffing foods and naming them was so intense that the moment I walked through the door, he would open his arms, run to me smiling, collapse into my hug, then demand, "Let's sniff!" He grew so attached to the activity—sticking his nose deep in a box of rice flour, crumbling the powdered hot chocolate in his fingers, tasting the dried currants in his hand—that he never wanted to do anything else. When my parents were visiting as well, they complained, "We want to see the boy!" Rightfully so—Elliott could have spent hours in the pantry, comparing the smell of cornstarch to that of apple cider vinegar. One day, my brother solved the dilemma. He gathered the most vivid-smelling foods on a tray, which he put down at Elliott's kid-size table in the living room. Elliott and I had been playing in his room when Andy came in and suggested: "Hey, Elliott, do you want to have a sniffing party?"

Elliott's eyes grew wide, and he stood up in anticipation. A look of amazement passed through him. "A 'niffing party!!" he shouted, and then ran into the living room.

I still say that to myself sometimes, when everything feels like it's going right. A 'niffing party! And when people offer me food, I don't stand by politely, nodding in approval like a measured adult. I tuck my hair behind my ears, then I duck down to put my nose just above the dish. I sniff. I inhale with my entire body, and I come up different. In moments like this, I feel as though I am simply living, not thinking or worrying or trying to impress. I am alive.

The fact is, we all have that amazement and play in us, somewhere. We could all still be little kids. We just believe that we have to be more contained when we are adults. No, thank you. As Picasso said, "Every child is an artist. The problem is how to remain an artist once he grows up."

Cooking is a creative act. When I'm stirring something in a pot, the smells wafting up to my nose, it feels the same as the pen drifting across the page. Deciding what to cook, then watching it emerge from underneath my hand, feels like something from the deepest part of me, and it will come out well only if I give it my concentrated awareness and relaxed joy.

Play with your food.

allow yourself to make mistakes

On my Web site, I display the most visually stunning photographs, the recipes I know will work when readers try to replicate them, and the stories with sentences I have honed into a rhythm that matches the one in my head.

Sometimes I think I make it all look too easy.

I have shared only the loveliest stories. I don't write about the days when I come home too exhausted to cook and simply sit on the couch, watching television, gnawing on the remnants of a roasted chicken from the night before. Or when I have a bowl of yogurt for dinner and go to bed early.

I take ten to twenty photographs for every one that turns out well. Sometimes it is fifty. Every good photographer does the same. Sometimes I have to make a dozen choices about light and composition and focus before that one snaps clear in the lens. Sometimes I take a good photograph, spontaneously, and then I take more just to be sure. In those cases, the first one is always the best. Every one of the blurry, boring photographs has taught me something.

I never feature the photographs of wilted salads, the soups that turned out just okay, the meat cooked too well to taste it anymore. When I first started playing with gluten-free cookies, I was horrified to find that the first batch out of the oven had spread, flubby and formless, like some of those strange creatures from Salvador Dali's painting *Persistence of Memory*. Furious tears rose to my eyes. "But I'm the baker!" I wanted to shout. And then I took a breath and went back. What could I do differently the next time?

Making mistakes is how I learn. I'm pretty sure it's how we all learn, actually. However, there seems to be some sort of national consensus that we should try to avoid as many mistakes as we can. When my students write poor first drafts, every one of them hands me the essay with a stiff arm and downcast eyes, ashamed. They look up, however, when I tell them, "Hey, it's your first draft. It's supposed to be imperfect." Then, we work together to make the next draft stronger, learning from the mistakes of the first draft.

Without mistakes, how would we learn?

There's a story my father told me when I was growing up. According to my father, the last words of Leonardo da Vinci were "What a pity it is that I have no more time left to learn." Now, when I started to research this tidbit as an adult, I find many sources citing his last words as, "I have offended God and mankind because my work did not reach the quality it should have." I hope not. That's such a sad, perfectionist way to go out. I think I prefer my father's story. My father's homily stuck with me, because it taught me that the most powerful motivating force should be to learn. I make a plethora of mistakes, every day, but the inexhaustible urge to learn, more and more, fuels me.

Here's the secret—find a way to allow the mistakes, while still laughing, and everything will start to taste better.

One winter day, I had a batch of report cards hanging over my head. What did I do about it? I decided to make a densely flavored, multistep mushroom soup, a re-creation of the vegetarian soup I made in my twenties.

The onions were caramelizing in my mighty stockpot. Shiitake and white mushrooms were searing in the skillet on the back burner. It was all coming together. I could feel it turning into food I'd want to eat. Perhaps I would write about it later. I began to write the piece in my head before I completed the task. In fact, I was so happy with the way this piece on mushroom soup would make me sound that I sort of forgot the soup itself.

Time to deglaze the pans. I reached into the refrigerator for the giant Tupperware container filled with the stock I had made the day before, and I turned toward the stove, still thinking of how brilliant that piece of writing will be . . . .

. . . and the container full of stock spilled from my hands. No, it tumbled. No, it rushed, danced, spinned, and then, *splat!* It crashed to the floor, the lid popped off (perhaps it wasn't on, really, and that's why it fell, but no matter), and mushroom stock splashed up. No, it fountained up. No, it surged, leapt, danced, and then spun. All over the kitchen. We're not talking a tiny spill. A little bobble. I mean, the entire floor was suddenly puddled in rich shiitake stock. My sheepskin slippers had dark splotches on them. My orange pants were a wet sienna. The coffee pot dripped brown. My face was splattered with stock. And, of course, the pan was deglazed, because there was stock all over the stove.

I paused for a moment, frozen in my spot. And then I started to laugh, as stock dripped down underneath my shirt. I started to giggle, and then I moved and almost slipped in the pool of brown liquid at my feet. I roared with laughter at my own near pratfall. The piece I had planned was blown out of my mind. I stood in the middle of the kitchen, dripping, stock gone, the morning possibly ruined, except it wasn't. I was laughing, in waves of giant giggles, then deep belly laughs. Waves of laughter, strong enough to knock down any of my remaining walls of resistance, anxiety, silliness, and worry.

I was fine.

And the soup? Well, I just used some leftover, gluten-free beef stock from a carton instead, and it tasted fantastic. I could taste the splattering of humility and the laughter in it.

For a moment, as I spooned the soup into my mouth, I mourned the loss of the brilliant piece of writing that would no longer be. And then I reminded myself, "That's all right. You're still learning."

I hope I always will be.

Cream of Mushroom Soup

This recipe doesn't require any mushroom stock, so you can't spill it on the floor. It's pretty fantastic, however. If you want to, you could spill some of it on the stove. I won't tell anyone.

3 tablespoons unsalted butter
2 tablespoons high-quality olive oil
5 cloves garlic, peeled and smashed
1½ pounds chopped white button mushrooms
1 large onion, peeled and diced
1 carrot, peeled and quartered
2 stalks celery, chopped
2 tablespoons chopped fresh thyme
3 tablespoons white rice flour
½ cup dry sherry
2 cups cream
2 teaspoons salt
2 teaspoons cracked black pepper

Sautéing the vegetables. Bring a stockpot to medium-high heat. Add 1 tablespoon of butter and the olive oil. Once the butter has melted and begins to bubble, add the smashed garlic cloves and stir for 1 to 2 minutes. Add the mushrooms, onion, carrot, and celery. Cook for 7 to 8 minutes, stirring occasionally to make sure the vegetables do not burn.

Adding more flavors. Add the thyme to the vegetables. Cook for 1 minute, or until the thyme starts to smell fragrant. Add the rice flour. Cook for 2 to 3 minutes, stirring frequently.

Splashing in sherry. Add the sherry to the mix. Continue to cook until the sherry has reduced in volume by half. When this has happened, cover the assembled vegetables and herbs with enough water to cover by 1 inch. Bring the liquid to a boil, then cook for 10 minutes on medium-high heat.

Finishing the soup. Puree the soup in a blender. Strain through a fine-mesh sieve and return the soup to the pot. Bring the soup to a boil. Add the cream. Whisk in the remaining 2 tablespoons of butter. Add the salt and pepper, taste, and serve.

Suggestions. This recipe is intended to create a thick soup, the right consistency for that green bean casserole you used to eat as a kid. If you would like to eat the soup at a thinner consistency, add some club soda to the soup when reheating it.

Feeds 6 to 8.

make the kitchen your space

When I first walked into the apartment in Seattle where I live now, wondering if I should rent it, I stepped into the open kitchen. I stood on the warm tile floor and spotted the light filling the space. I said yes before I had seen the rest of the apartment. I have never regretted that spontaneous decision.

After I regained my health, I started cleaning the kitchen. Rather than letting it be perpetually cluttered and thoughtlessly arranged, I deliberately made it my space. I printed photographs of memorable meals I had eaten over the years. I found spring green placemats, dishcloths the color of the swimming pool in summer, and crackled glass coasters for drinks.

Finally, I started haunting restaurant supply stores, where I bought a gleaming set of metal shelves—the same ones gourmet kitchen stores use to display their wares—for all my appliances and favorite new spices. In the late afternoon sun, everything shone. Of course, with all my supplies on display, cooking seemed even more enticing.

My kitchen isn't always clean, however. In magazines and the movies, kitchens are always enormous and gleaming. These photographs suggest that not only should we have the money for those convection ovens and slate countertops, we should also keep our kitchens as though we could all afford maids. Those advertisements make owners of actual kitchens feel bad, the same way fashion models make us feel as if we should spend all night sucking in our guts, hoping they will magically disappear when we wake up in the morning.

I eat. I cook. And I am imperfect.

One Saturday morning, I woke up to a messy kitchen. Since the last of my Friday night dinner party guests had left the house at 2 A.M., I had gone straight to bed. Oh, I had staved off sleep until I had scraped the biggest piles of food off the plates and put away all the perishable items. But I was exhausted, and I went to bed without loading the dishwasher.

When I woke up Saturday morning, I began brewing a pot of strong coffee and curled up with the paper, determined to clean for the rest of the morning. After all, I do prefer cooking in a kitchen that is clean to one that is cluttered with dishes. That was my intention—to clean all day long.

But the light falling through the skylights was so gorgeous that I had no choice but to take photographs. Liquid light spills down onto the table and white linoleum floor on sunny Seattle days. That morning, the light was so heartbreaking that instead of cleaning the kitchen, I pulled out every piece of food I had bought that week, placed it on my little table under the skylights, and photographed everything for my Web site. And in photographing those foods, I thought of four more recipes I wanted to try and had the photographs for all the essays on the Web site that week. If I had insisted on a tidy kitchen, I would have missed all that.

My friend Quinn came over that night, and there were still splatters on the stove when he entered the room. But we were making homemade potato chips; we were only going to mess it up again. Those chips tasted fantastic, and we laughed all night long. If I had let him in only once the kitchen was clean, we would not have shared that evening.

Dirty dishes? That's what comes from cooking full-course meals every day. Sometimes you just have to mess up the kitchen.

stock your kitchen well

Once I realized I needed new supplies and utensils because of the gluten, I looked around my kitchen and realized just how much I needed in general. Oh, I don't mean the novelty items displayed at the cash registers of luxury kitchen shops like avocado slicers, potato peelers that strap to the fingers, special napkin rings, or wineglass trinkets. No, thanks. I mean the necessary supplies of a real, working kitchen.

If advertisements in magazines are food porn, then gourmet kitchen stores are their purveyors. I've spent more time drooling in the fancy stores than I care to remember. You know the ones—the stores that sell colanders for eighty dollars because they come in tasteful colors. You don't need to shop at those stores to have a great kitchen.

The best and freshest ingredients are the key to great cooking. It does not matter what color your colander is. Focus on the food, and then find the items that will help you to make it better.

I like to shop at thrift stores. If you know of a good thrift store in your area, haunt it. A month after the winter holidays, or a few months after the wedding season is done, never-used appliances begin showing up. People buy expensive items like stick blenders or food processors and then find they never use them. Sheepishly, they dump them off at the nearest thrift store just so they can clear space in the cupboard for the next luxury item. I have found copper bowls for a dollar, a solid blender for three dollars, and a brand-new juicer for ten dollars. If you can breach your squeamishness about buying something used, you will find a treasure house of kitchen supplies at your local thrift store. I'm lucky enough to have a dozen restaurant-quality pots and pans—ten-inch skillets, crepe pans, stockpots, deep sauce-pans, and more—because my friend Brandon went on a mission at his local Goodwill to find me the best cooking supplies that twenty dollars could buy. I have used them every day for over a year, and they are better than the hundred-dollar skillet I bought the year before. I have a feeling that I will own them for another twenty years.

If you really want to feed your kitchen habit, start hanging out at restaurant supply stores. There are a plethora of items you may never need, like the plastic tortilla warmers, menu covers, and stainless steel hotel pans, but the basics of a good kitchen—such as metal spatulas, fine-mesh strainers, and large plastic cutting boards—are all waiting for you. I have loaded up an entire shopping cart with supplies I truly needed—including baking sheets, casserole dishes, rubber spatulas that will not melt in the heat, a citrus reamer, and mixing bowls—at my favorite restaurant supply store in Seattle, and l left the store with my wallet only one hundred dollars lighter.

You don't have to spend a lot of money to have a comfortable kitchen. The only thing that matters is that you create a kitchen space in which you will feel comfortable enough to sing and to play—and to make mistakes. Treat yourself to a new utensil every month. Have a little mad money set aside to buy a zester or a ricer for mashed potatoes. See what emerges from your kitchen with your new purchases.

invest in a good knife

Some items deserve their price tags. I simply couldn't live without my KitchenAid stand mixer, which was given to me as a Christmas present in 1994. Since then, it has whirled and swirled, mixing and combining cookies and cakes, now gluten-free, without once breaking down. I lug that heavy mass of a machine from my metal kitchen shelves nearly every day, and I bless its presence in my life. Indulge in something like that, and you will be sure to actually use it.

Even that is probably a luxury item, though. I could do without it, if I had to struggle through. There is one component of the kitchen upon which everyone should spend a little money, however, and that is a good knife.

I have a confession to make. For nearly a decade, I did all my cooking with a lousy twenty-dollar knife. I bought it when I was teaching at my little island high school and living in a prefabricated apartment behind the fire station. Living alone for the first time, I was thrilled to finally buy new supplies. So I bought a knife set at a giant discount store.

I shipped the biggest knife in my boxes to my apartment on the Upper West Side, when I moved to New York. In a city where I knew no one at first, opening the box with my kitchen supplies was what made me feel at home. I chopped vegetables, made stews by the dozens, and learned how to cook with truffle oil. Of course, so few people in New York City actually cook that my first roommates in that apartment were freaked out that I had such a big knife in the kitchen.

When I moved back to Seattle, I set up my kitchen again. I made basil goat cheese pasta on beds of arugula for the boyfriend at the time, along with slices of mango marinated in brown sugar and lime. I also enjoyed enormous salads, my first experience eating quinoa, and always, fabulous baked goods.

Through it all, I chopped with that same, flimsy knife. I never sharpened it. I couldn't even see my own reflection in it anymore. It was dull and barely worth the effort of picking it up. Dull knives are more dangerous than sharp ones.

Anyone else would have bought a good knife long before.

But good knives just seemed so darned expensive. Spending fifty to a hundred and fifty dollars for one knife felt like decadence. However, a few kitchen essentials make the entire experience worth it.

About six months after I learned that I cannot eat gluten, I decided to buy a truly great knife. I tried Japanese knives and German knives and locally made knives. I tried paring knives and cleavers and boning knives and bread knives. Then I picked up an eight-inch chef's knife.

It was like falling in love at first sight. I held it in my hand, and I never wanted it to leave. It just felt good. Heavy but not burdensome. Whole and solid and perfect. Holding it and then chopping some potatoes with it, I knew that I needed to own it. Why look further when you've already found it? I trusted my gut. I bought the knife.

I took it home and looked at it. Took pictures of it. Slid it in and out of its cover and listened to the swordlike *tzwing* sound it made when it emerged from its shell. At first, I didn't want to use it. It's so pretty. But then I broke that barrier and started chopping.

Here's a friendly warning for you, if you're planning on buying yourself a really good knife: respect the knife. When I started slicing vegetables, I was in awe of the knife. I've never chopped so slowly in my life. Everything simply fell into small slices and tender nibbles without the least bit of trouble from me. Eager to cut and chop and dice and slice, I took every vegetable I had in the house, and I watched it transform into magic under my hands. I was mindful and kind and alive.

But a few nights later, in trying to prepare for an impending party, I started making mushroom stock at 10:20 at night. The counters were covered with foods yet to be prepared. My large cutting board was yet to be washed. And I was in a hurry. So I started slicing onions, fast, on a small cutting board, precariously balanced on one of the stove's burners. Forgetting the knife's power, I used the same force I needed for my old one. Without a single second of warning, I took off a slice of the top of my ring finger.

Another lesson learned.

But let me tell you, the cut was worth it. I healed quickly. I will never take that beautiful knife for granted again, nor use it without being mindful. It is whisper sharp and gleaming in the dark night kitchen. I plan on owning this one for at least another decade.

recipes are only a rough guide

For months after my celiac diagnosis, I studied every good cookbook I could find with a fervent attention normally reserved for the work of scholars. After my study, I tried to replicate the vision I had formed in my mind on the plate. I am grateful for all that time trying to follow other people's minds, because it led me to mine.

These days, I'm cooking less often with recipes. More and more, I imagine a taste and then throw in ingredients that feel right. What happens if it all falls apart? Oh, well. It couldn't taste too terrible. Even if it does, I have a garbage disposal.

But I'm finding, again and again, that trusting the instincts I have developed from months of playing and making mistakes and feeding pleased people leads me to places I never knew existed. If I needed it all to be perfect, I'd be doing something else. It's the experimentation that I remember best.

The more I cook, the more comfortable I feel making up dishes based on the tastes of the moment. After leaning in every evening to smell what was bubbling away in the saucepan on the stove, I started to trust my palate.

Even the best recipes—including the ones in this book—are really only a rough estimate, like memories at their best. One of my Buddhist teachers in New York once told me that words are simply a finger, pointing out the path. And recipes? Yes, like that.

For example, I have given you the amounts for salt and pepper in all the recipes in this book where they are necessary. However, you should know that those are only the closest estimates I can make. When I first started cooking, I would have been a little frightened to see "a pinch of salt" or "a dash of pepper." Worse would have been "season to taste." But to be honest, after all this cooking, that's what I want to write now. Use the amounts I have given you as a guide and then decide on your own palate. Scrunch a bit of salt between your fingers and let it drift into the soup. Stir. And then taste. Is it enough? If not, try a little more. Play with it until you learn to trust your own tastes.

So feel free to experiment. Make your food by tastes and nibbles, not by the bible of recipes printed out in neat columns. Experiment in the kitchen, with the confidence of a child, alive to the possibilities and unafraid to make mistakes.

cultivate friends who love food

As the late author Laurie Colwin wrote, "No one who cooks, cooks alone. Even at her most solitary, a cook in the kitchen is surrounded by generations of cooks past, the advice and menus of cooks present, the wisdom of cookbook writers."

I once met a young woman in New York City, a thin, wan girl with no discernible personality. She sat next to me at an enormous table on the roof of a restaurant in the Village. Warm air blew off Sixth Avenue, and we were all delving into dishes of Mexican food. She sat with her hands in her lap. I thought perhaps she didn't have enough money for the check and quietly offered to help pay. She demurred.

"Becky doesn't like food," Sharon said to me, in between bites of her quesadilla.

"You don't like food!" I turned to this young woman.

"I don't know," she said as she twisted her hands in her lap. "I just don't understand why people talk about food all the time. It's just . . . food."

It was as though she were speaking moon-man language to me. Still, I struggled to understand. "Isn't there any food you enjoy more than others?" I asked her, hoping.

After a long moment of thinking, she said, "Cereal?"

We didn't talk the rest of the evening. I wasn't mad at her. We just didn't have anything to say to each other.

I don't understand people who don't love food. People who view food only as sustenance. People who don't moan when they eat mango ice cream with fig-ginger jam on top.

Almost every conversation I have with people I love eventually comes back to the food. One of the ways I became more comfortable in the kitchen is by gathering around me friends who adore food as much as I do. When I received the celiac diagnosis and found out I could eat only gluten-free foods, I knew that this would transform me, joyfully. Oh sure, there was an adjustment period, but it was brief. All I had to do was take down all my cookbooks from the shelf, research online, and start cooking. But mostly, all I had to do was call my friends. Friends who bring me organic potatoes from the farmers' markets, discuss recipes with me, introduce me to pomegranate molasses and great olive oil and new brands of dark chocolate, eat my meals with attention and grunting approval, and fill my e-mail inbox with encouragement and love and stories. They are my beloveds.

My memories of Sharon—my dearest friend since we were sixteen—include sudden stops for slices of rhubarb pie, citrus salmon with herbs in Seattle, steaming plates of pad thai with chicken, cider doughnuts, summer peaches, baked brie at New Year's, bowls of café au lait, and spare ribs that make us grin at each other through mouths stained with barbecue sauce.

Tita has been cooking for me for over fifteen years. The first summer I had to eat gluten-free, she made barbecue sauce by hand so we wouldn't have to rely on any bottled ones with lurking gluten. She still cooks out of a Wisconsin farm cookbook from the 1940s, and everything she makes tastes damned good.

Julie and I have traveled around the world and lived in several separate cities. Whenever one of us returns from travels, the first question we ask is "What was the most memorable meal?"

Amy loves cupcakes. If I want to make her happy, I find her photographs of cupcakes online. One part of my wedding present to her and her dear husband, Paul, was a T-shirt from Seattle's Cupcake Royale that read: LEGALIZE FROSTITUTION.

Pete loves going back home to Connecticut because he can walk into the butcher shop owned by old Italian men and buy a slice of a salami hanging from the ceiling.

Dorothy talks about Trader Joe's with the same obsessive fervency that I do. We compare dips and discuss the merits of buying mâche in bags. When she talks about food, she waves her hands in large circles in the air, and her voice speeds up.

Cindy grows quiet when she eats something spectacular, her eyes wide, her mouth not moving for a moment. And then she wants to talk about that bite for days after.

Jessica and I sit in her kitchen, up against the counter, facing each other, eating and talking our hearts out. We wax poetic about salads with twenty vegetables and lemon juice as the base of the dressing. The day after my horrible car accident, in which I nearly died, she brought me a bowl of chicken-noodle soup.

Once, Gabe told me that he had a childhood memory of being

in elementary school the day another kid had his birthday. After the treats were eaten, the boy's mom packed up the leftovers of the cake and smooshed them into a bag. Gabe always dreamed of that— eating cake out of a bag, the icing smeared to the top, soft bites emerging from the least gourmet of places. I teased him about this yearning—how weird is that?—but that night I baked him a cake and smashed it into a bag and then left it in his mailbox.

Mary has been baking bread for over fifty years. Even though she has never made a gluten-free loaf in her life, I'm sure she could figure out how. After a year and a half of bobbing together in Hydrofit, we still haven't made it through a class without talking about food. She brings me potato salad she makes from scratch early in the morning before we see each other. She's more alive than most of the thirty-year-olds I know, and I have to think that much of that is because her taste buds are still working so well.

All my friends have voracious appetites for life. Food is only the physical manifestation for the way we eat up our days, savoring the last tastes, and discussing them afterward.

making ceviche with merida

Merida makes noises when she eats, as I do. Not grunts or burps but little moans of appreciation.

When I asked her what she thought every person should have in his or her kitchen, she responded, vociferously, "Nobody should be allowed to cook in a kitchen for one. You cook with someone else. You cook with other people. You cook with your family. More than any other objects, that's what you need—other people." Luckily, I am rarely alone in my kitchen, because I can always invite Merida over to cook with me.

When her parents come to visit from New York City—her Ecuadorian father and her Dominican mother—they squish themselves into her tiny apartment kitchen and spend the entire afternoon making ceviche. It is, by the way, the best ceviche I have ever eaten.

Ecuadorian Shrimp Ceviche

3 pounds large prawns, tail and shell still on,
    cut and deveined
¼ cup kosher salt
1 fat heirloom tomato, diced
3 plum tomatoes, diced
juice of 4 lemons
juice of 2 navel oranges
1 medium yellow onion, peeled and minced
1 small red onion, peeled and minced
1 handful Italian parsley, chopped
3 tablespoons high-quality extra-virgin olive oil
1 teaspoon coarse sea salt
½ cup ketchup
3 cups freshly popped popcorn
Tabasco sauce (optional)

Preparing the prawns. Fill a huge pot with water and salt. Bring it to a rolling boil. Dump in the prawns. Cook the prawns until the moment they turn pink, which should be about 2 minutes. Allow them to cool and then shell the shrimp. Set them aside.

Making the marinade. Save 3 cups of the shrimp water and put it into a large bowl. Cool it in the refrigerator. When cooled, add all the other ingredients except the popcorn to the bowl and stir. Allow the mixture to sit for 15 minutes.

Tasting the marinade. Taste the ceviche. It should have a tomato taste, not a cocktail sauce taste. The texture should not be watery but not be chunky, either. It should have a cohesive consistency.

Combining all the ingredients. Put the shrimp into the bowl and join the two forces together. Put the bowl of ceviche in the refrigerator. Let it marinate overnight, which will make it taste phenomenal. (If you can't wait, let it marinate for at least 4 hours.)

Serving the ceviche. Put freshly popped popcorn at the bottom of a bowl and top it with the chilled ceviche. Add Tabasco sauce, if you wish. Serve immediately.

Feeds 4.

When I began my Web site, GlutenFreeGirl.com, I found a community of other friends: food bloggers. All around the world, thousands of food-obsessed people record what they eat, photograph their food, and rave about their favorite restaurants and recipes. Before I began my Web site, I really had no idea that such a community existed. I honestly thought I was only keeping my blog for my friends in far places. When people I had never met began leaving me comments—accolades for the way I explained gluten intolerance or questions about celiac disease, as well as compliments about my photographs and writing—I clicked on their names to find out who they were. This is how I met Shuna, from Eggbeater, a pastry chef from the Bay Area with a soft heart and a mean sense of what makes food sing. And Sam, from Becks and Posh, a British woman in San Francisco who seemed to know every great restaurant in town and still was gracious enough to introduce the world to all the food bloggers she admired. I met dozens of people this way, through their Web sites. I read Clotilde's site, Chocolate and Zucchini, checking back regularly for her pithy evocations of life as a young woman devoted to great food in France. I read David Lebovitz's site devotedly, every day, coming back for his explorations of chocolate and Paris. Heidi at 101 Cookbooks stunned me with her gorgeous photographs every time I saw her site. Luisa answered burning questions for me—Is the recipe the *New York Times* printed today worth making?—by cooking from the food sections of major newspapers at The Wednesday Chef. The Amateur Gourmet, This Little Piglet, Chez Pim—they all drew me in and made me feel as though I was privy to their lives.

And increasingly with some of these bloggers, the comments on one another's posts became personal e-mails, chatty letters back and forth between friends, even if we were friends who had never met. I had pen pals who loved to write about their meals. In some instances, I even met some of these food bloggers in person, and they all confirmed what I already knew from reading their pieces: these are funny, alive people, voracious and expansive, curious and kind. Luisa and I had cups of thick hot chocolate at the City Bakery in New York, and we started our conversation running, as though we had known each other for years. Jen from Prepare to Meet Your Bakerina joined us, charmed us both, and made this an official food bloggers gathering.

Then there is Molly. Molly writes one of the best food Web sites in the world: Orangette. For months, I had been slurping up her words, reveling in her stories and wanting to meet her. Every time I read her site, ideas bloomed in my mind, ideas for exquisite dishes I could create to feed my friends. Afterward we'd all raise our forks to the sky in her honor.

She had seen my site as well. She wrote to me, and I wrote back. For days, we wrote feasting e-mails to each other, chatty and filled with food descriptions. It wasn't long before we met for cups of spicy chai, then a walk through late-summer sunlight at the Ballard Market.

She sampled from the bruschetta stand that I had been wanting to try for months, the one that compiles all the freshest foods from the local stands surrounding it, then creates tiny bites on crisp bread. Obviously, it's off my list, but I had looked at it longingly as I walked by it each week. Molly tried a sampler of three, including the octopus offering. As we sat on a little bench, life bustling walking by, the light falling at our feet, she bit into one bruschetta and made a little moan. I knew in that moment that we'd be friends.

I am moved, all the time, by the people who have entered my life through my Web site and through my love of food. The thousands of readers I have met through my blog—the ones who write to thank me, to ask me questions, and to share their own stories—inspire me to cook more and more. They have become an integral part of my life.

It doesn't take much for two people to come together. Dip forks in bowls together and talk about the luscious taste of food—we are connected. My friends are fairly different from one another, but they all share an absurd laughter, tender hearts, a keen sensitivity, and a hungering curiosity about the world. They all love food.

So, if you don't have friends who love food, find some. Life is more bountiful with those people around.

12

life,
gluten-free

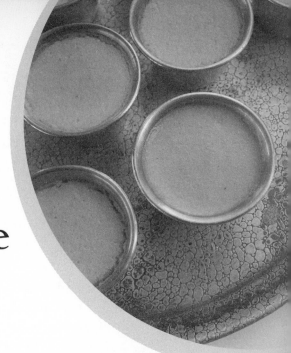

In February 2006—ten months after I was diagnosed with celiac disease—I got my first tattoo. Surrounded by friends, I sat waiting for a man with ink-festooned arms to leave his mark on me. I had in mind a simple design, a design so simple that the East Village professional was annoyed because he had so little to do. In small, plain letters, on the top of my left wrist, I had *yes* permanently inked onto my skin.

Why? So many reasons. I wanted it placed there so I could look at that word instead of a watch. Whenever we look at our watches, we are saying no. *I want to be somewhere else. Oh boy, I'm late. I wish this would end.* These are all ways of denying the moment as it exists.

I felt a shift happening in my life. All throughout my childhood, I heard no. Now, after knowing my own story and cooking gluten-free food, spontaneously everything in my life pointed toward yes.

Just a month before, I had finished my first book proposal and sent it off to New York, hoping a fabulous literary agent would like it well enough to sign me. I had been writing essays on my Web site for nine months, and I was waiting for something to be born.

I had been writing all my life. As soon as I learned to read, I wanted to write. As soon as I knew that human beings created books, I wanted to write one. Over the past thirty-nine years, I had read thousands of books. I had filled countless journals, from childish ones with beige paper and teddy bears in the corners to expensive ones lined with quotes about writing to thick black artist sketchbooks with plain paper. Personal essays, short stories, bad poems, dense analyses of Baudrillard's take on Disneyland—I have written them all. When asked why I write, I have no other answer than "I have to breathe."

One of my dear friends dubbed me Seymour years ago, because of a quote from J. D. Salinger's book, *Seymour: An Introduction.* When asked to respond to his brother Buddy's short stories, Seymour responds with the following response: "Were most of your stars out? Were you writing your heart out?"

For those past nine months, I had been writing my heart out on my Web site. I had been writing about my joys, my favorite tastes, my discoveries, and my love for food and life. So many people had entered my life through my Web site, and through my love of food. I have kept my Web site for the joy of it and because I have felt I am helping other people directly. I never in my life imagined that it would lead to what has been handed to me.

Since I went gluten-free and joyfully embraced my food fate, my life has grown larger and more passionate, hilarious and touching by turns. There have been countless dinner parties with friends. New people whom I had met through their food Web sites have become dear to me. In the winter, after I wrote a funny little paean to the tiny Le Creuset pot I had purchased, someone arranged to have the Le Creuset company send me an entire set of its cookware for free. I had made friends with chefs and people who owned a gourmet kitchen store and others who led chocolate tours of Paris. No longer did I feel like that frightened kid who sat alone in her room.

Around the New Year, my Web site won a Food Blog Award for Best Food Blog in the World with a Theme. I could hardly believe the life that had arrived, especially when the act of writing every day felt like reward enough. I woke up every morning with a feeling of curiosity about what awaited me next. I felt alive. I said yes.

As much as I had loved teaching, I knew it was time to leave it soon. I wanted to jump into the world of being a full-time writer. I didn't know the way there, but I knew I wanted to go. Teaching meant a steady paycheck, health insurance, and a retirement fund. Writing meant all of those would be stripped away. Fear said to stay where it was safe. My gut said what my life wanted. I wanted to say yes.

So I had *yes* tattooed on my wrist.

Unequivocally, I said yes to every part of my life. But to dating? I was ready to say no to dating. At age thirty-nine, my fortieth year loomed large. A late bloomer, I perpetually felt behind the rest of society. After I turned thirty, I hit the dating world with a dedicated passion. Online dating, friends of friends, men I met in restaurants—I tried my darndest. Certainly, I have stories of brief loving relationships and horrendous blind dates both. However, I just couldn't seem to find anyone to match me. The entire process exhausted me. After the car accident, I focused on healing and feeling alive. After my celiac diagnosis, it seemed my energies were going elsewhere—into writing, into food, into helping people through both of these means. I was ready to throw away the possibility of ever finding someone to marry.

In fact, the previous August, on my thirty-ninth birthday, I had sent out an e-mail announcing my three-day, fortieth birthday party the next year. I called it "To Hell with the Wedding Party." Since I couldn't seem to meet anyone right for me—and I remained joyfully aware of how lucky I was to be alive—I decided to give up on that elusive search for the mate. Hell with it. Who needs a wedding to bring all my friends from around the world together? Maybe I would just marry myself.

However, after my trip to New York, I decided to open myself to it, one more time. Several friends of mine there looked resplendently happy with partners they had met through online dating. Even in the bitter cold, I noticed couples walking down the streets of Manhattan and felt jealous. And at the core of me, there is always hope.

So I remembered the end of Molly Bloom's soliloquy, the last line of James Joyce's *Ulysses*, a book so important to me I had read it four times. Thinking of her husband, with whom she has been struggling, Molly Bloom remembers again when they met, and how Leopold asked her to go out with him. She responded, in her mind, with, ". . . and yes I said yes I will *yes.*"

I had *yes* tattooed on my wrist. I went home, I signed up for an online dating site, and I tried again.

I put up a profile the day I returned home from New York, with the following headline: "I'll make roast chicken, garlic mashed potatoes, and flourless chocolate torte. You do the dishes. We'll dance in the kitchen." To my surprise, I was flooded with responses. Write about food, and the men come calling. But the problem was, they all turned out to be disappointments. There were cups of coffee and glasses of wine with men who didn't know how to laugh, or who weren't really alive or interested in food, or men who seemed interested but turned out to be confused. It felt the same as the times I had tried online dating before: strange and untenable. One man even wrote to me, after a volley of interesting e-mails, upon finding out that I cannot eat gluten: "I'm sorry. You seem great, but I really love bread, and I just can't imagine dating someone who cannot eat wheat." Oh, my. After six weeks of trying this—and finally hearing from the literary agent that she wanted to sign me—I decided to devote my energies to my writing. Who needed this? I gave up. I vowed to never look again. I told myself that I was saying yes to my writing instead, but really, I just quit.

When I told the dating site to not renew my subscription—thank you—they informed me that I still had five grace days left. *Who cares?* I thought. They're all going to be the same. I vowed to not even look at the e-mails piling up in that account. But curiosity grabbed me the day before my subscription ran out. I flicked through all the people who had sent out requests, and even felt a small tug of self-satisfaction that I had made the right choice. No, no, no, no . . . Wait.

Something in his eyes looked familiar. I was tempted. But I was done dating. I had promised myself—no more of this. I sat in front of the computer, looking at his picture, my hand hovering over the mouse of my computer. Should I? I clicked on the rest of his profile and found out that he was a professional chef in a well-respected restaurant. I remembered Merida telling me about a meal she ate there: "The food was tremendous." *Damn.* Well, now I had to answer. But I expected nothing. I sent a little "wink" back, imagining that I would not hear from him. I felt ready for my dating days to finally be over.

To my surprise, he sent me an e-mail the same day, with his real e-mail address within it. (The dating service uses a double-blind function, so you never see each other's real e-mail address.) If he had not sent it to me that day, I would never have met him, since my subscription was about to expire. And his e-mail had only one question: "If a man was to prepare a meal for you, what would you consider the ideal meal?"

That was hard to resist. So, in spite of my resolve, I sent him this answer: "Honestly, it would be this: one he made with love. With his own hands. In season, beautifully seasoned. Made to connect, every taste an experience, meant to be eaten mindfully. Surprising tastes. Wholly unexpected and familiar at the same time. It would taste of laughter."

He wrote back, and we started writing to each other about food, pouring out our favorite tastes and memories from childhood and places to eat. I kept my guard up—after all, I was done, right?—but he kept knocking it down.

Within the first couple of days, I sent him the address to my Web site. And frankly, I did it to ward him off. Too many men had read my site and been intimidated by my passions and the length of the essays. I expected him to be the same. But he grabbed my attention when he wrote a long e-mail to me telling me how much he loved my writing and my enthusiasm for food. And the one post he remarked on? The essay I had written for my nephew's third birthday.

And so, we finally met. I walked into one of my favorite coffee shops, prepared to be disappointed. When we saw each other, we both recognized the other. I sat at a table, working on a piece of writing for my Web site, content to let him come to me. Why didn't I jump up to say hello and start the conversation? I felt relaxed with him in the room, already. After standing in line and waiting for his grande latte, he moved to the station with the sugar and milk. At this point, I moved toward him, to finally say something. I looked at the glass container of sugar in his hand, pouring a white stream into his milky coffee, for at least thirty seconds. Without hesitating—or even saying hello, really—I slapped him on the arm and said, "Hey, do you want some coffee with your sugar?"

And immediately afterward, I thought two things: "God, that was rude, Shauna. And oh damn—I just hit him on the arm, so now he knows I like him." And immediately afterward, he thought, "Oh God, she's a smart-ass. I love it."

On the first sunny Seattle day that spring, we enjoyed some free wine and our second date. We meandered through the wine tasting, slowly, laughing and talking. An hour and a half later—after telling me how much he loved reading my Web site—he leaned over and kissed me. We ran across the street, holding hands, skipping in the sunlight, suddenly children together, happy and laughing. At Union, we ate perfectly sautéed branzino, some gorgeous soft cheese with fig marmalade, and dishes of some fabulous food. I don't remember those dishes because he kept leaning in for kisses, playful and affectionate, with his hand on my leg.

We walked up the Harbor Steps, holding hands, in the moonlight, kissing at every new level. He walked me to my bus stop, and he held me. He didn't hug me. He held me. And he said, breathlessly, "You taste like truffles."

"But I haven't eaten any truffles," I said. "I never have."

"Oh, we'll have to take care of that," he told me. We both grinned.

On our third date, we spent the afternoon at Pike Place Market, where he bought me tulips, and I bought grapes, and we fed each other triple cream cheese off the ends of our fingers, as we sat in the park. From that day onward, we talked every day, he calling me from his restaurant to tell me what he was cooking that night, me telling him stories from school and what I had written that day. We never really dated. We just started our life together. There were no games, no veneer, no wondering or hesitation. We just started loving each other.

We went to cheese festivals, ate brunch at French restaurants, looked at food magazines together, walked downtown holding hands, and stopped at every restaurant to look at the menus of the day. We cooked dinner together and ate languorous breakfasts on the weekends. We made plans to cook stocks and make salsa and shop at the farmers' markets all summer long. We woke up in each other's arms, happy and warm. We spent the morning listening to the Beatles, drinking coffee with our legs intertwined as the sunshine fell through the blinds. We looked at menus online of restaurants we love and wondered what they were cooking that day. We danced to songs that instantly became ours. And we did dishes in each other's kitchens after three-course meals we had made together. We were food geeks, goony in love.

After two weeks of this, we uttered "I love you" into the darkness above us at the same time.

You see, in one of those rare twists of fate that yields only happiness, after the most spectacular year of my life, I was given more. The most spectacular *yes* of all: real love.

We had both fallen in love at first sight. Call us ridiculous romantics if you want. We don't care. We know. When we began talking, we felt like friends. Sure, there was enormous physical attraction, but that was not the deepest flavor. Instead, we tasted comfort. We laughed, mostly. We slipped into conversations like sliding into warm water, and we haven't left yet.

Talking with him felt like keeping my hand wrapped around a warm cup of coffee. That conversation tasted like potato-leek soup, like apple crisp, like coq au vin just out of the oven. We wafted vanilla and sugar between us. We devoured each other's words, and every one of them felt like *yes*.

And when he hugged me at the end of our first date, I almost started crying. It felt that good. He held me, his arms strong around me, pressing me into him. And in that moment, I honestly felt all the loving that would follow, all the days together, all the laughter. That moment is when I said *yes* to him.

Late in the evening, the Chef comes to my house, after an entire day of cooking at his restaurant. He smells of warmth and richness, the mingled scents of grilled lamb, Spanish goat cheese, and Rainier cherry ice cream. When I kiss him, I can taste everything he made that night. He tastes of great food and hard work and real love.

Some nights, I cook for him. After all, he rarely eats a home-cooked meal. He simply sips and nibbles on bits of food in the tiny kitchen where he's producing meals for other people. And most people are too intimidated to cook for him. Hell, I'm intimidated, too, because I am nothing but a passionate amateur in comparison to this man. But, then again, he doesn't really write—we love the fact that we have different talents. He adores the pieces I write, and I adore the food he feeds me. So I don't need to be great when I cook for him. I cook with love, and he eats, happily. And then, after much coaxing from me, he gives me notes on how to make it better.

But most nights, to my astonishment, the Chef insists on cooking for us. With great enthusiasm and a confidence I wish I could know in my body, he throws together something delicious for us to eat: warm salads, grilled fish, potato purees, or eggs scrambled with sautéed zucchini and smoked salmon. When I protest that he shouldn't have to work when he has been cooking all day, he looks over his shoulder at me as he stands at the stove, and says, "I'm cooking dinner for the woman I love. This isn't work."

And so I sit at the table in the little kitchen nook, my feet propped up on the kitchen counter, regaling him with stories and grinning at him, adoring him.

The Chef had a rigorous training in traditional French cuisine at the New England Culinary Institute, and he has been cooking all his adult life in great restaurants in New York, Colorado, and Seattle. However, when he cooks in my kitchen—quickly becoming his kitchen—he enjoys simple food. He cooks foods that are perfectly seasoned and in season, but simple, nonetheless. These are foods that a mother might make—apple dumplings, roast beef, or chicken potpies.

The first time the Chef was in my kitchen, we cooked together. We stood in front of the stove and talked, both our hands chopping vegetables, the rhythm of our conversation matching the rhythm of our knives. He ate my roast chicken and ran from one end of the kitchen to the other side of the living room, whooping and hollering at the taste of it, then stopping to do a jig on the kitchen floor. I ate his mashed potatoes with roasted yellow peppers and yelled out a little hallelujah. We danced together.

Rosemary-Lemon Roast Chicken

1 lemon
10 to 12 skewers of fresh rosemary
10 garlic cloves
zest of 2 lemons
1 teaspoon sea salt
½ cup high-quality extra-virgin olive oil
1 whole chicken, about 4 pounds, cleaned and cleared of giblets

Preparing. Preheat the oven to 500 degrees F. Bring a pan of water to boil. Once the water is boiling, add the lemon. Let it bob around in the water for about 5 minutes. While the lemon is boiling, dunk the rosemary skewers in the boiling water for 1 second. The hot water will release the essential oils in the rosemary, yielding more flavor. Strip the skewers of the rosemary needles. Put a large roasting pan into the oven and heat to sizzling.

Making the paste. Put the rosemary, garlic cloves, lemon zest, and sea salt in a large mortar. Using your arm strength and a pestle, grind all the herbs and ingredients together for a few moments, until you have a gorgeous, green-yellow paste. Add the olive oil and stir the mixture about for a bit. Take a whiff.

Prepping the chicken. Using your hands, smear the rosemary-garlic-olive oil paste all around the chicken. Make sure to tuck under the drumsticks, as well. Caress all of it onto the skin. Put the chicken in the heated roasting pan, back side down.

Before you slide the chicken into the oven, retrieve the hot lemon from the boiling water. Place it in the cavity of the chicken, tucking it down as far as it will go. If it is a large lemon, you can cut it in half and slide each half down the cavity. (Putting a hot lemon into the chicken—instead of a cold one, as most of us have done—releases the juices of the lemon immediately, which will infuse the chicken throughout the cooking process.)

Roasting the chicken. Slide the roasting pan into the oven. Cook the chicken for 15 minutes. (Don't worry if the oven starts to smoke a bit. That's natural.)

Lower the heat to 425 degrees F and cook the chicken until the internal temperature in the chicken's breast is 155 degrees F and the drumstick has reached 180 degrees F on your meat thermometer. This will probably take about 45 minutes, depending on your oven.

Finishing the chicken. When the chicken is done, pull it out of the oven and let it rest for a few minutes before you carve it. You should have the juiciest, easiest roast chicken you have ever made.

Serves 4.

The next time he came over, on his day off, the Chef stood in my kitchen and made me a meal. Simply watching him chop the blanched tomatoes fascinated me. I had been wielding my expensive sharp knife for months, but it sits better in his hands. I felt sloppy in comparison. But that encouraged me, too, because I have so much to learn about food and how to create it. He's teaching me, every day. Seeing him chop anything entices me to wander over closer and watch his technique. Sometimes, I lean down as he is finely mincing garlic and take in a whiff, of spiciness and familiar warmth, clarity and head rush, and I love him even more.

When he starts to really cook, we don't talk. We have music on in the background. The sun is shining through the skylights. I might do some dishes behind him, in a futile attempt to keep the kitchen clean. But mostly, I just sit and watch him, as he bends over and listens to the food in the skillet. He pinches salt between his fingers and dashes in far less than I would, until the flavors start to sing. He pays attention, deeply, to the textures and colors and smells and flavors, a little smile upon his lips. He plates up our food, his face wide with excitement, because he knows how much I'm going to love what he has made with his hands.

In the morning, the Chef and I sit at the kitchen table and concoct recipes. I have to admit—I adore being part of a couple that loves food. Never in my life, not even in my most daring dreams, could I imagine feeling this comfortable in the kitchen with a man. Two cups of coffee, the remnants of breakfast between us, and my pen darting across the page of my notebook, full of food notes—we are completely absorbed in each other and the process.

And what we have found, over and over again, is that food is foreplay, food is fuel for our relationship, food is one of the languages we speak together. When we visit spice stores, his eyes grow wide as he asks me to smell Vietnamese cinnamon, then puts a bit on his lips and tells me to kiss him. I taste its warmth and my eyes grow wide. While most people regard going to the grocery store together as drudgery, we linger in every aisle and sniff everything we can. We shop with our arms around each other, hands tucked into the other's back pockets. We only remove them to grab something else from the shelf.

We are a couple everywhere we go, but where we are most alive is in the kitchen, in the morning, after being together all night. Sleepy and happy, we stumble in for coffee and sit down to talk about food. The morning after he made me a spectacular gluten-free veal goulash, we had leftovers for breakfast. Let me tell you—oh, my god. *Yes.*

This is a man who knows how much his seventy-nine-year-old father loves tomatoes, so he sends heirlooms to him in Tucson by FedEx during the summer. This is a man who always makes sure that my cup is full of hot coffee. This is a man who makes potato-leek soup with wild truffle honey at his restaurant, saying that he thought of me when he made it, then spoons some into my mouth and I cry, because it is the best soup I have ever eaten. This is a man who has a stack of pink Post-it Notes filled with all the different variations of mashed potatoes he wants to make. This is a man who makes the finest mashed potatoes I have ever eaten in my life. This is a man who eats three bowls of my Moroccan lentil soup. This is a man who calls me from his restaurant to tell me, in excited tones, about the basil oil he made that afternoon from the Thai basil we bought at the market that morning, and how he swirled the dark green liquid through the chilled tomato soup he made just after. This is a man who never makes me feel like the rank amateur that I am, but who says he will teach me everything he knows.

There is, of course, so much more to him than his food. He is, truly, the sweetest man I have ever met. But food is central to him, as it is central to me. Spending all day living in his senses—chopping onions, making veal stock, dreaming up soups and fish specials for hours at a time—makes him practical and alive. He doesn't think too much. He just greets the day as it arrives to him. I never thought

I'd meet a man like this. He is, without question, a sensualist, alive to his senses and living in his body. (I will say no more on that matter. But—*yes*.) As he told me within a couple weeks of meeting me, the reason he has been cooking in restaurants since he was thirteen years old is that in making food, he can give people such joy.

He brings this joy not only to me but to all who eat his food. He is the sole chef at a small restaurant here in Seattle called Impromptu Bistro. This intimate place, with twenty-five seats and windows overlooking Lake Washington, is based around the impeccably chosen wines. Every three months, the restaurant changes the region of the world from which the wines come. And then, the Chef creates an entire menu and cooks all the meals, from start to finish, every day. There are few chefs who can do this: maintain a relationship with the food producers, shop at the farmers' markets, choose the cheeses, make the stocks and soups, create all the appetizers, grill and sauté the entrées, and concoct the desserts. After my first night of eating there, I was amazed.

He had a table by the window reserved for my friend Traca and me. Every member of the staff had heard about me, so they all smiled when I said, "Hi, I'm Shauna." On the table sat a vase full of purple tulips. Stephanie, the waitress, said, "The Chef bought those for you." *Oh.* And in the arrangement, little squiggles of pea shoots, which he had bought at the farmers' market with me that morning. I noticed his attentiveness. He had the waitresses send over two glasses of sparking wine, then a bottle of red wine. And then, a cheese platter, with three of the most delicious cheeses I have ever eaten: a young, soft pecorino, unlike anything else; a Pierre Robert, which melted on touching my tongue; a California goat cheese, threaded through with ash, with a light, clean taste. I was in tears. My friend couldn't speak for the pleasure.

Next, came a polenta terrine, studded with roasted asparagus and topped with seared foie gras. For the entrées, the Chef sent out a perfectly cooked beef tenderloin, rare, on top of blue-cheese mashed potatoes, with a port-balsamic reduction sauce. Better yet, he had called the cheese producer to ensure that the cheese was gluten-free.

Alongside all this was a perfectly grilled piece of rockfish, with kala-mata olives and a bacon vinaigrette. It took everything I had to not lick both plates clean.

After the entrées, I told the waitress to go back to the kitchen and tell the Chef I said one word: joy. I looked up a minute later to see him standing in the doorway, smiling wide at me, arms thrust in the air. Then he started jumping up and down like a little kid.

For dessert, there was a polenta cake with lemon syrup. And freshly made strawberry sorbet, which he had made just for me. How could I not love this man?

How could I not say yes?

Wonderfully, beautifully, I have a restaurant now where I *know* I can eat gluten-free and not worry about cross-contamination. The Chef is impeccably careful about it, teaching everyone at the restaurant how to take care of me. Once it became known that his restaurant was safe for those who need to eat gluten-free—through my Web site and the message boards—people came flocking in, to eat his food and to catch a glimpse of the Chef. Most of them come to thank him at the end of the meal, in tears, grateful for the first res-taurant meal they have eaten in years.

Without my noticing, the Chef started creating more gluten-free entrées. Always excited by food, he loved watching the look on my face when I first ate his halibut baked in banana leaves or seared lamb chops with garlic terrine. In the first two months we were dat-ing, I jumped in my seat when I saw two or three items I could eat on the menu.

Within three months, I could eat everything there. He made his entire restaurant gluten-free, for me.

The Chef began to think like me. When he dreamed of crab cakes in Dungeness season, he naturally thought of bread crumbs made with the sorghum bread I had invented. When he made those crab cakes with a shrimp mousse and paired them with avocado-cabbage slaw, jicama, and saffron rice, no one in the restaurant knew this was a "special diet" menu. It was simply great food.

I knew, however. I knew that he eliminated wheat flour from his kitchen. I knew that he cleaned everything meticulously to avoid cross-contamination. I knew that he began making tart shells with gluten-free dough and dredging his fish in rice flour before pan searing it.

He has told me that he loves this, that he is learning an entire new world of food. He had never heard of amaranth or teff before reading my Web site. Now he dances with them in the kitchen.

But I love this grand gesture of his more than I could ever say. What kind of man makes an entire restaurant gluten-free to feed his love? The Chef. When someone asks him why he did it, he always says the same thing, "I don't want to make any food that she can't taste. She's my muse."

This means that every one of you reading, those of you who must be gluten-free—you now know of one restaurant where you can eat safely.

The Chef is, without a doubt, tenderly aware of what will and will not make me sick. After I educated him a bit about gluten, he never made an issue of it. He has certainly never made me feel odd because I cannot eat wheat. Once, while we were eating a spectacular meal at one of our favorite restaurants in Seattle, kissing each other over the table, he did something that knocked me out. We had ordered a duck breast dish, with duck confit, asparagus, and potato gnocchi. He asked for the potato gnocchi to be put on a side plate, so it couldn't touch my food. We had also ordered a grapefruit margarita, and we were sipping it between us. Halfway through the meal, I was prattling on about something happily, telling a story to my new love. I reached for the straw and nearly put my lips upon it. The Chef grabbed my hand, gently, and said, "Nope. I just drank from that, after eating the gnocchi. Don't touch the straw. I don't want you sick." I drank from the side of the glass instead, and gulped back my tears. It's amazing how a gesture like that can make me feel loved. This man, this Chef, he takes care of me, beautifully.

One early afternoon, in the middle of working on this book, I wandered back into the tiny kitchen of the Chef's restaurant in the afternoon. Something warm and enticing drew me in, something besides the promise of kisses. It smelled oddly familiar in there. I had to know.

When I walked in, I saw him, grinning, that little-boy enthusiasm in his eyes. In his hands? A loaf of warm bread—crusty, yeasty homemade bread. He held out the red terrine pan to me, so that I could bend down my head and smell. When I lifted my eyes to him, he saw the tears in them.

"Sweetie, what is it?" he said, his face a sudden scrim of worry.

I couldn't talk for a moment. Then, I gulped out, "You made me bread."

The Chef infused this particular loaf of bread with dried lavender. Later, he made lavender toasts and topped them with smoked salmon mousse he made himself. I dined off that for days.

A week later, I went to the restaurant to have dinner with a friend. As she and I chattered and drank wine, Deb put down a basket of bread between us. I didn't even look at it. I'm used to blocking that out. However, Deb turned toward me, and said, "The Chef sent that out for you." I folded back the white napkin and saw it: slices of warm, crusty bread, for dipping in olive oil. Gluten-free.

I nearly cried again.

Once, someone asked him how he could make his entire restaurant gluten-free. How did he change his French-inspired cuisine to never use flour or wheat? What he said, immediately, was this: "You meet this woman. You hold her in your arms. You fall in love with her. And then you find out that there's something in your food that makes her sick. You teach yourself to adapt."

One evening, at home, he made us gluten-free pizza. On top were roasted orange and yellow peppers, caramelized onions, fresh mozzarella, rosemary, and a decadent treat—an heirloom tomato out of season. The crust was chewy with a familiar bounce against the teeth; dense and yeasty; a willing sopper for the olive oil soaking into it. The bottom held an unexpected crunch, only unexpected because no gluten-free pizza crust, in my experience, ever has that shattered-by-the-teeth bottom, the crisp and crackle of a truly great pizza. This one did. It tasted like pizza. No, it tasted like truly great pizza.

When I thanked him, I saw his face—blurred through my tears— soften. And he said, "I don't want you to feel any different because you have celiac disease. I want to be able to make you any food you want, and have it taste the way you want. It may take a while to make some of them right, but I'm going to do it. Because I want to feed you."

If you want to understand just how much I love this man, let me share this fact. In my kitchen, there is a drawer next to the stove containing a cutting board and a loaf of bread. And in the refrigerator is a six-pack of beer. For an entire year, not a single speck of gluten entered this house. But as soon as the Chef entered my life, I decided to let gluten back in the house, too. He is meticulous about using only that cutting board, then wiping down the counters, when he eats bread. And when he does eat bread, or drinks a beer, he refrains from kissing me until he has brushed his teeth. Having to wait—and knowing that he is taking care of me—only makes me want to kiss him more.

Besides, it is his house now, too.

When we spent our first long weekend together—the both of us free from work for a few days—we already knew we had years ahead of us. What was the rush to say what we would do next when we knew? Why not sway with the taste of what we were experiencing instead?

The weekend was glorious, in the most mundane way. We went on long walks. We read the Sunday paper in bed. We went grocery shopping, which always excites us. We watched the *South Park* movie and episodes of *M.A.S.H.* We talked and danced and laughed. For days, I cooked for him, since he cooks for ten hours a day at work. He was patient. He was truly grateful for my split pea soup and fresh crab and scrambled eggs. I watched his eyes close in pleasure, and I felt more gratified than I ever had after finishing any piece I have ever written.

However, by Monday night, he could no longer stand it. "I'm going to cook for you," he said. When I protested that I wanted him to not have to work, he said, "This is not work. I want to cook for you. Sit down and watch." So I did. I watched him chop up slices of bacon into tiny pieces, all of them even. I watched him sauté and whisk and mix and wilt. I watched him lean back and dance with a skillet, as he tossed the food without a spatula. (Oh boy, that impresses me.) I watched him wind his way through our meal, smiling.

There was a piece of pork tenderloin, wrapped in bacon and sprigs of rosemary, seared fast then thrown in the hot oven. But honestly, neither of us paid too much attention to that. Instead, the Chef kept saying, "Wait until you try this salad." He was making a traditional French salad, minus the croutons, with frisée, bacon, and a poached egg. He asked me to sit down on the couch and wait. I did.

When the plate arrived before me, the spidery frisée sitting crouched on the plate, the poached egg glistening and jiggly, and the indescribable smell of warm bacon vinaigrette wafting up toward me—warm and rich and touched with vinegar—I nearly fainted. He grinned as I moaned at the smell of it. We sat back and relaxed.

And then I took my first bite.

It tasted like Paris, my first taste of freedom, walking down the Champs-Élysées. It tasted like childhood, with the sharp taste of smoked bacon. It tasted like comforting Sunday mornings, with the poached eggs. A bite of vinegar, a crunch of pale greens, a richness of mustard, a depth of something I couldn't quite name. It tasted like the life between us, and everything yet to come.

"Oh f—," I spluttered, then I looked over to see the Chef beaming at the sight of me enjoying his food.

Without planning it or thinking about the consequences of the question I was about to ask, I said with urgency, and a hint of irritation that it had taken me this long, "Would you just move in with me?"

Tears formed in his eyes, then he said, "Okay. Of course I will."

And so, he did.

And then my fortieth birthday arrived. Some of my dearest friends in the world—including Merida and Sharon, Gabe and Monica—gathered at the Chef's restaurant for a Friday night dinner. That night was a small gathering, just my closest friends, and the Chef cooking for us. We laugh on the patio, in the twilight air, then lean down together over the food. After the first bite, everyone stops talking. Prawns with scallions and a garlic-almond puree. Pork tenderloin stuffed with chorizo sausage, brined for days in cloves and sugar, then roasted, accompanied by saffron risotto and an organic heirloom tomato sauce. Lamb chops dusted with cumin and coriander, alongside roasted eggplant and a cucumber yogurt sauce. Braised black and white beans with a warm bacon vinaigrette and fried sage leaves. Chocolate mousse with amaretto.

When the Chef comes out to see us all, Merida nods at him, raising her fork toward him. She doesn't need to say a word for him to understand how she feels.

Gabe turns toward him and says, "This is extraordinary food. It feels so personal and direct. I feel like you made this just for me." The Chef grins, happily, and nods at him. That's how he makes his food.

Sharon looks up at the Chef and points to the remnants of the garlic-almond puree on her plate, and says, "Could you just make me a vat of this so I could swim in it and eat my way out?"

The laughter rings out toward the dark night sky and the lake beyond us.

I couldn't imagine a more beautiful birthday celebration, my dearest friends in the world with me, and the man I love more dearly than I ever imagined I could, making us this food.

As I sat writing one of the chapters of this book, trying to describe the taste of great olive oil, the Chef plopped down a tray of butternut squash flans. This metal tray, tested in his oven a hundred dozen times, was burnished and crackled. It felt ancient.

When I saw them, I oohed and said, "Oh, can I have one?" He smiled, because he loves how much I love his food. But—no. They were for the restaurant. He was trying out the first batch for his new menu, a monthly revelation.

I admired the smooth surfaces, noted the cracked ones, and grabbed the camera. The light falling through the large windows felt so urgently vivid. I captured them in the light, which was almost like eating one.

A few weeks later, I turned to him in his little restaurant kitchen, and said, "You know, you still haven't given me any of that flan." He nodded and smiled his slow grin at me. Before he started serving it, he had tweaked the recipe three times. After he started cooking the menu, he did four more variations before he was happy with the flan. Even though he had been serving it, and all the plates had come back clean, he would not let me eat one until those flans were *done*.

Finally, it was time.

He prepared an order for me. He ran a hot knife around the edges of the flan, tipped the little metal cup onto a clean white plate, and flipped the plate over. After a solid thwack, he turned the plate up toward the light. There it was—a perfect flan, solid and just a bit jiggly. Around it, he placed toasted pecans, then drizzled some of his sherry gastrique. The plate passed toward me.

I sat on the patio, under the heat lamp, alone in the glimmering light of twilight. My fork dove in.

Softness. Warmth. Full taste of butternut squash, the quintessential taste of autumn. Slightly sweet. Something pungent, wonderfully smooth. The taste escaped down the sides of my tongue.

I dipped the next bite in the sherry gastrique, dark brown and drizzled. It tasted of roasted onions, somehow, even though there were no onions in it. "That's the caramelization," he told me, hovering at my shoulder, watching for my reactions. The sharp bite of vinegar, the yielding kindness of sugar. All of it dancing in my mouth.

I leaned up my face to kiss him in the darkness. He grinned and walked back to the kitchen.

I turned, once more, to my plate.

If anyone tells you that living gluten-free is deprivation, tell that person to change his or her mind. It's just being alive.

epilogue

yes

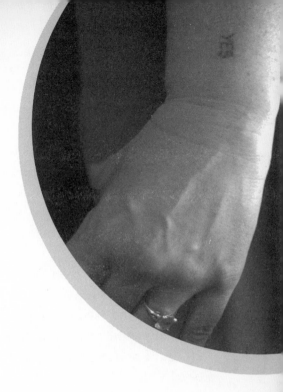

The most urgent reason I wanted that tattoo in February? I didn't admit it to anyone else at the time. It felt private, a little silly, and all mine. But still, my reason was there. It had been since I was fifteen, when I first became a Beatles fan.

The story goes that when John Lennon first met Yoko Ono, he met her at one of her art shows. As he toured around the strange white shapes, he came upon a ladder in the corner. At the top of the ladder, the ceiling. On the ceiling, a magnifying glass dangling down. As he climbed up the ladder, he expected to see something in the magnifying glass like STOP THE WAR, or FUCK YOU. He expected it to be incendiary. Instead, when he reached the top of the ladder and peered through the magnifying glass, he read, in teeny tiny letters, YES.

He climbed down the ladder and went to meet the artist. Apparently, they spent the entire night talking, two soul mates finally meeting each other. At dawn, they ate a bowl of cereal and kissed. They were in love. They never stopped.

When I was fifteen and first read this love story, I thought, "I want one of those!" As I grew older, I grew more jaded about love at

253

first sight, but some part of me still believed. I still wanted it. Relationships waxed and waned, but none of them felt right. I was still looking for someone who said yes.

And so, when I thought about getting the tattoo, I thought of this story again. As silly as it sounds—and it even seemed so to me—I wanted to mark myself with that love story. I thought, "If he is out there, somewhere, that man who's going to love me fully, he will recognize me when he sees this. He will know this story, and he will know."

On our first date, the Chef noticed my tattoo. I didn't know it at the time. On our third date, as we sat in a park outside Pike Place Market, feeding each other and kissing, he held my wrist and asked me, "Tell me the story about this." I started to say all the many reasons. But I noticed that I didn't want to tell him the John and Yoko story. I wanted him to know it first.

After I had run out of all the other reasons, I started, slowly, "And then there's this story about John Lennon—"

"And Yoko Ono?" he said.

Startled, I couldn't talk for a moment.

"You mean the ladder story," he told me. I nodded.

I told him the story, even though it was clear he knew it. When I finished with ". . . they finally kissed, and they were in love," he looked at me with tears in his eyes. And then he leaned in for a long kiss.

Oh yeah. All right. Boy, you're going to be in my dreams tonight.

On the first night we spent together, he looked at me and said, "Now it's time for you to see my tattoo."

Puzzled, I said, "You have a tattoo?"

He nodded, and then he slowly took off his shirt. On his upper arm, he had a tattoo of John Lennon. He got it when he was twenty-two.

I just stared at him. "You have John Lennon on your arm," I kept saying. "You have John Lennon on your arm."

"And you have Yoko on yours," he told me.

That was when I *knew*. That long phase of my life—of not feeling well and wondering at my place in life and being alone—was finally done. And the next one, equally long, if not longer—of feeling alive and knowing where I belong and loving this man—had just begun.

For the last half hour, he had been calling me, repeatedly. "Hurry up!" he mock shouted over the phone.

"Sweetie, we can't go any faster. The traffic is terrible." My mother laughed as she drove, and my father smiled so hard his cheeks grew red.

We were headed to the Chef's restaurant. My parents and I laughed and talked, in easy tones and decades-of-history familiarity. After a childhood of fighting and Wonder bread, now there was peace and good food. With enormous persistence, a thousand honest conversations, and more forgiveness than I could have imagined feeling when I was in my twenties, we had healed our relationship. I always joked with them: "You two have really grown up well."

Now, we were parking in front of the Chef's restaurant.

They settled into the table by the window, the one always reserved for me. While they surveyed the lake and smiled to themselves about the occasion, I went back to the kitchen to see the Chef. I found him, short of breath and sweating. Hortensia, his feisty dishwasher, and I flapped kitchen towels at him, to calm him down. "Sweetie pie, it's okay," I told him. "Breathe."

My parents knew why we were there. They had met him weeks before and adored him, immediately. He knew that they knew why we were there. There was no surprise to any of this. Still, he was so palpably shaking with nervousness that I had to hold him close and stroke his hair to calm him down.

I went back to the table and grinned at my parents. Telling them how nervous he was, I asked them to be patient. "Look, this might seem a little hokey, but it's important to him."

My mother grabbed my hand and said, "Shauna, it doesn't seem hokey to me at all." My father already had tears in his eyes.

The Chef emerged from the kitchen, his hands shaking, a little.

Everyone hugged, then I held his hand as he sat down at the table across from me. Still too nervous to say what he needed to say, he asked about their days and made small talk. He hates small talk. I nudged his foot under the table. "Go ahead," I whispered at him. My mother smiled.

I had been so nervous for him, in anticipation, that somehow I had not been able to take in the beauty of what was about to happen. When it happened, I felt it in my gut.

I watched him say, to my parents, "Mr. and Mrs. James, I love your daughter with all my heart. She is the most amazing woman I have ever met, and I promise to take care of her for the rest of her life." I started to sob. I couldn't help it. I was prepared to find this lovely, but I had no idea I would feel this grateful. The man I love was asking my parents for their permission to marry me.

My mother reached across the table to grab his hands, and said, "Of course, Danny. Of course. We can't think of anything better."

My father looked at him, deadpan, and said, "Ah, no." When the Chef's face looked stricken for a moment, my father softened immediately and said, "Oh, Danny, nothing could make us any happier." My father gave my love a big hug. The Chef relaxed. Everyone laughed. And then the Chef walked back to the kitchen to make us our meals.

It was, without a doubt, the best meal my parents had ever eaten. That eight-course Italian meal my father recounted all through our childhood? It paled in comparison to this one, he swore. My mother, suddenly more daring for the happiness of the moment, actually took a bite of my father's beef, done medium rare. "Oh, that really does taste better," she said, and I smiled. They looked fulfilled. All those years before this one? They fell away in that moment. We were simply eating, and alive. The food is what connected us.

And the food? It was familiar and wholly unexpected at the same time. Beautifully seasoned, local, and in season. Made with his own hands. Every mouthful a mindful experience. Honest. It tasted of laughter. It was made with love.

Yes.

what is gluten and where does it hide?

Gluten is the elastic protein in wheat, rye, and barley (as well as triticale, spelt, durum, and semolina). This particular protein makes pizza crust chewy, fills baguettes with those pockets of air, and keeps puff pastries light and crunchy. Gluten helps bread dough to rise and gives baked goods the familiar mouthfeel that compels people to buy muffins in the middle of the afternoon.

It seems impossible, at first, to imagine living without gluten.

Living gluten-free is not as simple as avoiding those foods that obviously contain gluten. Gluten can hide in places one might never suspect. Soy sauce? Contains wheat. Root beer? Malt flavoring from barley. Almost every kind of licorice? Made with wheat flour. Even lipstick can be made with wheat as a binder. Every time you lick your lips, you are growing sick. Gluten, it seems, is everywhere.

After the Food Labeling Act of 2004 went into effect in 2006, reading food labels became a bit easier for those who must eat gluten-free. Now, anything containing wheat (or processed in a facility that uses wheat) must be labeled as such. However, food producers are not required to label the foods that contain gluten. At least not yet. Therefore, gluten can hide in a number of ways and in places people might not expect, such as the following:

- malt flavoring (from barley)
- hydrolyzed vegetable protein
- MSG made outside the United States
- natural flavors (this could be anything; you have to ask the food producer)
- caramel coloring made outside the United States
- dextrins (especially in vitamin supplements and prescription medications)
- wheat starch (in the United States and Canada; in Europe, wheat starch is allowed)

Confused? Sure. Living gluten-free means being mindful every time you take a bite of food or put on lipstick. There is no question: living gluten-free is a way of living, every hour of the day. But in a life without gluten, there is freedom.

For a guide to gluten-free flours and how to use them, please visit glutenfreegirl.com.

resources

support resources

Where do you turn if you are gluten-free?

Celiac.com
P.O. Box 279
Gardena, CA 90248
www.celiac.com

Celiac Disease Center at Columbia University
Harkness Pavilion
180 Fort Washington Avenue, Suite 934
New York, NY 10032
(212) 342-4529
www.celiacdiseasecenter.org

Gluten Intolerance Group
31214 124th Avenue SE
Auburn, WA 98092-3667
(253) 833-6655
www.gluten.net

National Foundation for Celiac Awareness
124 South Maple Street, 2nd Floor
Ambler, PA 19002
www.celiaccentral.org

University of Maryland Center for Celiac
20 Penn Street, Room S303B
Baltimore, MD 21201
(800) 492-5538
www.celiaccenter.org

gluten-free food producers

Some of my favorite gluten-free food producers.

Bob's Red Mill
5209 SE International Way
Milwaukie, OR 97222
(800) 349-2173
www.bobsredmill.com

Crave Bakery
(415) 826-7187
cravebakery.com

The Cravings Place
568 NE Savannah Drive, Suite 5
Bend, OR 97701
(541) 388-BAKE (2253)
www.thecravingsplace.com

Ener-G Foods
5960 First Avenue South
P.O. Box 84487
Seattle, WA 98124-5787
(800) 331-5222
www.ener-g.com

Gluten-Free Mall
4927 Sonoma Highway, Suite C1
Santa Rosa, CA 95409
(800) 986-2705 (order line)
www.glutenfreemall.com

Mona's Gluten-Free
13422 NE 177th Place
Woodinville, WA 98072
(866) 486-0701
www.madebymona.com

The Teff Company
(888) 822-2221
www.teffco.com

WOW Bakery
WOW Baking Company
8314 Greenwood Avenue North #1100
Seattle, WA 98103
(206) 816-5200
www.wowbaking.com

food blogs

Food blogs mentioned in this book that are well worth visiting.

101 Cookbooks
www.101cookbooks.com
Heidi Swanson takes stunning photographs of the food she creates: vegetarian, organic, and succulent.

Becks and Posh
www.becksposhnosh.blogspot.com
Sam Breach has an insatiable curiosity for all things food. A British woman who loves a French man, she explores San Francisco for all things gustatory.

Chocolate and Zucchini
www.chocolateandzucchini.com
Clotilde Dousulier has a puckish sense of humor and an unfailing interest in procuring the best foods in Paris and offering them to us.

David Lebovitz
www.davidlebovitz.com
Besides being the former pastry chef at Chez Panisse—and thus an incredible source of knowledge for all things sweet—David is a wonderful guide to Paris, where he lives.

Orangette
www.orangette.blogspot.com
Molly writes eloquently—with a touch of devilish humor—about the simple

pleasures of food and her life in Seattle, with her husband, Brandon, whom she met through her blog.

Prepare to Meet Your Bakerina
www.bakerina.com
Jen writes about baked goods, life in Queens, and politics with a sweet, snarky sense of humor and a keen eye for detail.

Tea and Cookies
www.teaandcookies.blogspot.com
Tea, who lives in the Bay Area, writes beautifully about eating locally, eating through the challenge of food allergies, and her life with food.

The Wednesday Chef
www.wednesdaychef.typepad.com
Luisa has an unfailingly good eye for what makes a recipe. Thank goodness she spares us the rest of the trouble of making some of the recipes featured in the Wednesday food sections of the nation's major newspapers.

cooking resources

These places will make you a better cook.

Chef Shop
1415 Elliot Avenue West
Seattle, WA 98119
(800) 596-0885
www.Chefshop.com
This is an exquisite resource for all the finest ingredients worth splurging on. Tim and Eliza, who run the company, introduced me to Sorrento Lemon olive oil, organic honey from Hawaii, and Moroccan spice rubs. Click onto their Web site and you will be absorbed for hours.

Cook's Thesaurus
www.foodsubs.com
This is an endlessly fascinating encyclopedia of a Web site, with photographs and explanations of nearly every food in existence.

Le Creuset
www.lecreuset.com
This company makes some of the finest cookware in the world.

Seasonal Cornucopia
www.seasonalcornucopia.com
Run by an organic chef in Seattle, this Web site is an exhaustive resource for seasonality.

Sur la Table
www.surlatable.com
This place is dangerous for those who love to cook. Try not to buy something.

World Spice Merchants
1509 Western Avenue
Seattle, WA 98101
(206) 682-7274
www.worldspice.com
Whole and exotic spices from around the world make this store a singular sensory experience.

food shopping and eating in seattle

If you live in Seattle or are planning to visit, check out the following.

A & J Meats
2401 Queen Anne Avenue North
Seattle, WA 98109
(206) 284-3885
Charming, old-fashioned, and unfailingly kind—this is a great butcher shop.

Don and Joe's Meats
85 Pike Street
Seattle, WA 98101-2085
(206) 682-7670
These guys have been selling great meat in the Pike Place Market for decades. Trust them.

Palace Kitchen
2030 Fifth Avenue
Seattle, WA 98121
(206) 448-2001
www.tomdouglas.com/palace
One of my favorite restaurants in Seattle. I have always eaten safely here.

Pike Place Market
85 Pike Street
Seattle, WA 98101
(206) 682-7453
www.pikeplacemarket.org
If you visit Seattle and don't visit the dozens of stalls and little corners of the Pike Place Market, well, then you didn't visit Seattle.

Puget Sound Consumers' Co-op
600 North 34th Street
Seattle, WA 98103
(206) 632-6811
www.pccnaturalmarkets.com
Puget Consumers' Co-op is one of the best co-ops in the country, with its attention to local, organic, and compassionately grown food.

Seattle Neighborhood Farmers' Market Association
Northeast 50th Street and University Way
Seattle, WA 98105
www.seattlefarmersmarkets.org
Farmers' markets dot the city, but my favorite is the one in the University District on Saturdays.

University Seafood and Poultry Market
1317 Northeast 47th Street
Seattle, WA 98105
(206) 632-3700
Old-fashioned and not needing to change, this tiny spot has the best seafood in town.

Uwajimaya
600 5th Avenue South
Seattle, WA 98104
(206) 624-6248
www.uwajimaya.com
For any Asian food you could desire, this vast market will take hours of your life, joyfully.

Volterra
5411 Ballard Avenue Northwest
Seattle, WA 98107
(206) 789-5100
www.volterrarestaurant.com
Truly remarkable Tuscan food. Don (the chef) and Michelle (the manager) are wonderful people who fell in love in Italy, then returned to Seattle to open this restaurant. They also understand gluten-free concerns entirely.

Impromptu Bistro
4235 E. Madison Street
Seattle, WA 98112
(206) 860-1569
www.impromptuwinebar.com
If you would like to eat at the Chef's restaurant, he would love to feed you.

index

DATE DUE

FEB 0 2 2008	MAY 1 8 2009
MAR 2 2 2008	
MAR 2 6 2008	SEP 1 4 2010
APR 0 1 2008	
JUN 0 5 2008	
JUN 2 8 2008	
JUL 3 1 2008	
MAR 0 4 2009	
JUL 3 0 2009	
SEP 2 1 2009	
JAN 0 4	

BRODART Cat. No. 23-221